UNIVERSITY OF
WOLVERHAMPTON

DEVELOPING YOUR CAREER IN NURSING

WITHDRAWN

D0540973

WP 2017957

Also available from Cassell:

Chellen: *Information Technology for the Caring Professions*

Chellen: *Word for Windows for the Caring Professions*

Chellen: *Excel for the Caring Professions*

Mayho: *Positive Carers: rights and responsibilities of HIV positive health care workers*

DEVELOPING YOUR CAREER IN NURSING

Edited by
Robert Newell

UNIVERSITY OF WOLVERHAMPTON
LIBRARY

Acc No. 2017857

CLASS
610.
73069
DEV

CONTROL
0304332267

DATE 12 JUL 1996

SITE NEW

WV

CASSELL

Cassell
Wellington House
125 Strand
London WC2R 0BB

215 Park Avenue South
New York
NY 10003, USA

© Robert Newell 1995

All rights reserved. No part of this publication may be reproduced
or transmitted in any form or by any means, electronic or mechanical, including photocopying, recording or any information storage
or retrieval system, without prior permission in writing from the
publisher.

First published 1995

British Library Cataloguing-in-Publication Data
A catalogue record for this book is available from the British
Library.

Library of Congress Cataloging-in-Publication Data
Developing your career in nursing / edited by Robert Newell.
    p.   cm.
    Includes bibliographical references and index.
    ISBN 0–304–33226–7 (hb).—ISBN 0–304–33228–3 (pb)
    1. Nursing—Vocational guidance—Great Britain.   2.
    Nursing—Vocational guidance.   I.   Newell, Robert,
    1954– .   [DNLM: 1. Nursing.   2.   Career Mobility.
    3.   Career Choice.   WY 16
    D4892 1996]
    RT82.D47 1996
    610.73'06'9—dc20
    DNLM/DLC
    for Library of Congress   95–11758
                                                                  CIP

ISBN: 0–304–33226–7 (hb)
       0–304–33228–3 (pb)

Typeset by Action Typesetting Ltd, Gloucester
Printed and bound in Great Britain by Biddles Ltd,
Guildford & King's Lynn

CONTENTS

LIST OF CONTRIBUTORS

Sandra Baulcomb, BA, RGN, RM, NDNCert, DN, Cert Ed
Lecturer in Nursing, Institute of Nursing Studies, Hull University

Peter Birchenall, MA, PhD, RNMH, RGN, Dip Nursing, RNT
Principal Lecturer in Health and Nursing, University of Humberside

Margaret Clarke, BSc, MPhil, SRN, ONC, RNT
Emeritus Professor of Nursing, Hull University

Peter Draper, BSC, PhD, RGN, RNT Cardio-thoracic Nursing
Certificate (ENB 249)
Lecturer, Institute of Nursing Studies, Hull University

Bob Gates, BEd, MSc, RMN, RNMH, RNT, Cert Ed, Dip N
Lecturer, Institute of Nursing Studies, Hull University

David Justham, BSc, MSc, RGN, OHNC, RNT
Lecturer, Institute of Nursing Studies, Hull University

Robert Newell, BSc, RGN, RMN, RNT, Dip N Ed
Lecturer in Nursing, Hull University

Caroline Plews, BA, MA, RGN HVCert, RNT, PGCE(A)
Lecturer in Nursing, Institute of Nursing Studies, Hull University

Lesley Sheldon, BSc, RGN, RSCN, Dip N Ed, RNT, Cert Public
Policy
Lecturer in Paediatric Nursing, St Bartholomew's Hospital College of Nursing

Rachel Tucker, BA, RGN
Research Co-ordinator, Department of Public Health and Epidemiology, University College, London

Linda Veitch, BSc, RGN, RCNT, NBS Critical Care, NBS Neuro-medical/Neurosurgical
Lecturer in Critical Care Nursing, Institute of Nursing Studies, Hull University

SECTION 1
DECIDING TO BE A NURSE

Nursing is about people who care for others, and about people who need caring for. This book is for those who think that a career in nursing might be for them, and so it's probably true that you think of yourself as a caring person. The book is written *by* nurses, with those who want to *become* nurses in mind, so all of us have been through the process of deciding to **become** a nurse. Despite all the changes in nursing over the years, some of which you may have heard about, and some of which this book talks about, we still think that nursing is an incredibly worthwhile activity, both in terms of the service it offers others and in terms of our personal satisfaction.

We do realize, though, that the decision to become a nurse is not one to be taken lightly, and we also appreciate that there are a number of hoops to be gone through between making that decision and actually starting to nurse. So this book has been written with the aims both of guiding you through the different educational routes you can take to achieve that end and of helping you to make up your mind about whether to train as a nurse at all. It is because of this that we not only describe the various ways in which nurses are educated in this country, but also try, with the aid of examples from nursing practice, to sketch out what you can expect to happen after qualifying as a nurse. The diagram on page 3 shows the possible career routes through nursing, right from application through qualification and future career. We hope that, at the end of this book, you will still want to be a nurse – hopefully more so than when you began to read it. Most of all, however, we hope we will have helped you in reaching the best decision for yourself for the future.

In the first chapter I talk about the work of nursing, and set out some of the arguments for and against being a nurse. Perhaps you will have heard some of these before. Many of them are repeated by nurses wherever they meet and are, in a sense, as much a part of nursing culture as the jobs we do, the shifts we work and the clothes we wear. If you don't know any nurses personally, this chapter tries to give you some 'instant experience' of what nursing is likely to be all about.

A note on gender

With the exception of some of the case history material, we use the female personal pronoun throughout, as a reflection of nursing as a predominantly female profession and of women as the greater consumers of health care.

A PATHWAY THROUGH NURSING

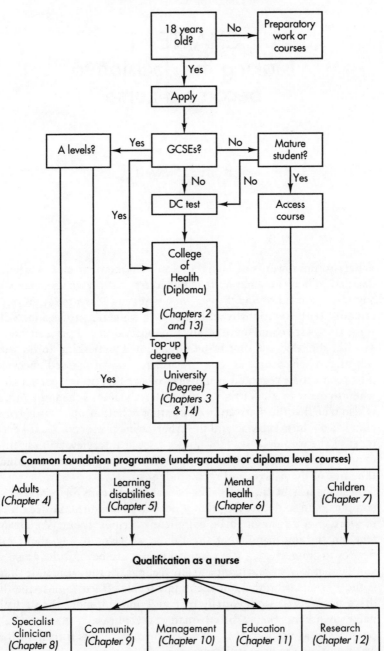

CHAPTER 1
Making the decision to become a nurse

Robert Newell

What are the rewards of being a nurse? I remember clearly when I decided to become a nurse. It is not likely that my experience is in any way typical. For one thing I am a man; and, even today, nursing remains, both traditionally and actually, a women's profession. Still, some things are common to us all, and most nurses, if pressed would say, like me, that wanting to be a nurse had something to do with wanting to help people or look after them. I say 'if pressed', because it has come to be regarded as unusual to have that desire, particularly when so many jobs offer far greater material benefits than nursing. It is also true that the motivation of wanting to help people has become almost a cliché in nursing and the other caring professions. However, most of the would-be student nurses I see at interview will say this, or some variant of it. My colleagues and nursing friends say much the same of themselves and their students.

Perhaps it is because this idea of wanting to care for people is so complex, and so deeply felt, that it becomes both difficult to express in words, and difficult to be completely serious about. We always feel, on the one hand, that the things we want to say about our desires to connect with other human beings are beyond the grasp of words, that we can't do justice to our feelings. At the same time there is the apprehension that our seemingly feeble efforts to describe the drive to care will seem equally trite and, indeed, more than a little naive to others. So we often qualify the phrase 'I want to help people' by saying 'I know it sounds corny but . . . ' as if to show that we appreciate the dangers here.

There's no need to do this. Our feelings are no less deep because we lack the words, and no less legitimate because others have felt them, or have expressed them more fluently. The desire to care for each other is basic to humanity, even to its very survival. John Donne says: 'Any man's death diminishes me, because I am involved with Mankind.'[1] This involvement in and with humanity is what nursing is all about, and just as each person's death can diminish us, so each life can enrich us. This joy and pain in life often finds great expression in the life of a nurse, because we see people at the 'great' times in their lives – great happiness, great sadness, great strength. It may be that here we see each other at our most human. For me, it is this chance to share with others that is the essence of nursing, and which underpins the many tasks which nurses undertake with and for their patients. It is also, I believe, nursing's chief reward.

I am not going to talk at any length about the history of nursing, because this book is much more concerned with the here-and-now of becoming a nurse. Nevertheless, it cannot be denied that nursing exists within a tradition, at least in British culture. Much of this tradition is extremely positive, emphasizing and encapsulating the best characteristics of people, in the way I have suggested above. In another sense, however, the history of nursing is a history of servitude. Both of these aspects make a part of what nursing is today; let's examine them in a little more detail.

SAINT, MARTYR, SERVANT?

Given the sorts of values I ascribed to the desire to care, it is hardly surprising that religious orders have, in the past, contributed a great deal to nursing. Indeed, it was a major task of many holy orders, most especially nuns, to minister to the sick, and there remain many predominantly nursing orders today. From one point of view this is fine, but consider the fact that in the past becoming a nun often represented the best of a tiny range of alternatives for a woman, particularly one who was not considered marriageable, and certainly one of the few jobs in which a woman could rise to the very top, gain respect and wield authority over others. In the convent, so in nursing; and nursing, like many other institutions has had its share of restrictions, rituals, formal and informal laws of conduct.

Many of the paternalistic restrictions placed on the nurse in earlier years have gone, but three things remain areas of difficulty. First, nursing is, at least in this country, considerably dominated by medicine in many of the settings in which it is practised. Second, nursing is still regarded by many as a profession suitable only for women. Finally, nursing is still struggling to find an independent voice in health care. Indeed, many have argued that this final issue reflects the broader struggle of women to find a source of power in society as a whole.

Balanced against these difficulties, and a gradual encroachment of men into the higher levels of the profession, nurses have striven hard to develop their independence. There are now many areas in nursing which do not rely on medicine, and we shall be looking at some of these in later sections of this book. Nursing is losing its image as a vocational occupation requiring chiefly the ability to perform personal services for others, and associated principally with male views as to the best attributes of women. Likewise nurses, particularly senior nurses, are no longer content to fill a role of servitude to other professions, but increasingly become involved in decision-making about policy at the highest level. The struggle for independence as nurses is far from over, but this in itself makes it an exciting time to enter nursing, since many great changes are now going on.

THE SCOPE OF NURSING

Although a great many nurses continue to work in hospital settings, providing care for patients in ways which would be readily recognized by members of the public as nursing, large numbers have also taken a far wider role, involving work in the community, and in the promotion of health and preventative care, rather than simply working with sick people. This shift towards health as a major concern of the nurse is true whether the nurse is working in nursing adults, children, people with mental health problems or people with learning disabilities (mental handicap). So, all these nurses are likely to be involved in working to promote health and prevent illness or relapse, as well as working with those who are currently defined as 'sick'. This has greatly increased the scope of nursing as a profession, and nurses can be found working in a variety of settings, with a wide range of client groups. The sections of this book devoted to working and progressing as a nurse deal with many of these special settings and disciplines in detail, but at the start of your consideration of nursing as a career, it is worth remembering that the traditional view of nurses working with physically ill people in hospital wards, as a kind of doctor's assistant, presents a very distorted view of nursing. In fact, as a trained nurse, you will have the opportunity to work in outpatients' departments, GP clinics, theatres, occupational health departments, clients' homes, and many other settings. Many aspects of nursing, for instance health visiting, midwifery, stoma therapy require the nurse to act with virtual or complete independence from medical practitioners. If we also examine the work of the children's nurse, the psychiatric nurse and the nurse for the mentally handicapped, then the scope of nursing is even further widened, and the newly qualified nurse is faced with an almost bewildering array of choices in further career pathways.

As with the perception of the role of the nurse, so in the scope of nursing great changes are in progress. The whole health care system in the UK is changing. Whilst controversy rages over the appropriateness of these changes, and many people considering nursing will have already formed their opinions about this, there can be no doubt that two issues will dominate such debates: the reorganization of provision of care away from hospitals and into the community, and the provision of care along 'market forces' principles. Both these principles are already altering the way in which nursing and nurse education are carried out. Nurses are increasingly responsible for organizing a service and retaining responsibility not only for clinical, but also budgetary implications of what they do, whilst attempting to ensure both quality and value for money for the clients whom they serve, within the often stringent funding constraints which apply. In community provision, it seems likely that eventually only a minority of nurses will work within traditional hospital settings, with the rest being in the community, working in clients' own homes, social service facilities, GP practices, nurse-led health centres and mental health centres, small 'community hospitals' and the private sector.

QUALITIES AND SKILLS OF THE NURSE

I spoke earlier about the nature of nursing as a caring profession, and the impetus to care for others which propels many people into training as a nurse. Is it essential to be a 'caring' person to be a nurse? Almost certainly it is, but almost every person is caring; it is simply that some wish to demonstrate their care for others in the context of their daily work, and to develop further that side of themselves. If this is a side of us which we wish to develop, then nursing offers the opportunity to do just that. However, it also carries the potential risk of losing contact with that caring part, as the undoubted stresses and strains of working very closely with distressed people take their toll on the new nurse. It used to be the case that student nurses were counselled against becoming 'involved' with patients and clients, and an air of professional detachment was encouraged. By and large, nurse educators now recognize that nurses will form close bonds with their patients; indeed, I suggested earlier that this may well be what nursing is all about. As a result, if the nurse is to remain open to the needs of her patients, she needs not only to be able to form these bonds, but also to be sufficiently resilient to cope with the emotional pressure that sharing deep and often traumatic personal experiences with others brings. In the best of nursing education, trained nurses and nurse educators help, guide and support the student through the process of finding out how to combine sensitivity to others with the ability to withstand the demands that sensitivity makes on themselves.

As well as the kind of mental strength I am hinting at above, there is no doubt that nurses need to be physically fit. We exert a powerful influence over our patients, who are often looking to us as an example of what constitutes healthy living. For this reason, as well as our own wellbeing, it is important for nurses to be able to appreciate and look after their own health needs. More practically, nursing is often hard physical work, and so self-care is all important. Finally, nursing combines this physical work with an increasingly rigorous educational programme, either to degree or diploma level. As well as considerable intelligence, student nurses need to be alert in order to make the best of acquiring and applying this intellectual knowledge, and good health is required for this. This is not to say, however, that people with disabilities cannot enter and be successful in nursing. The issue I raise here concerns fitness, and many people with disabilities are at least as fit as those described as able bodied.

To return to the issue of intelligence: happily, the days when nurses were required merely to carry out a pre-planned set of instructions, usually decided upon by a doctor, have now passed. The struggle for independence of action as a nurse continues, but nurses have gained considerable clinical freedom in determining their own actions in their dealings with patients. As a consequence, the concepts of the nurse as accountable for her actions, and as a 'knowledgeable doer', are now at the core of the profession. These ideas mean that the trained nurse is required to be able to give an account of *why* she performed a particular action when giving patient care, including offering, where applicable, an examination of complicated theoretical material which could be taken to support her actions. This requires considerable depth of understanding.

More practically, nurses are now intimately involved in the education of their clients and patients during health and illness. In order to offer *effective* education, the nurse requires a great deal of personal knowledge of the subject matter she is seeking to share with the public. It must be remembered that, as a student nurse, you will be required to take aboard this theoretical knowledge in the context not only of maturing as an individual, as all students must, but also whilst undertaking practical work that is both physically and emotionally demanding, and therefore a potentially formidable distraction from application to study.

Nursing also requires the mastery of a considerable number of complex practical skills. Some nurses are drawn towards the so-called 'high-tech' environments of operating theatres, critical care units and accident and emergency departments. Certainly this is highly skilled work, but nurses in other areas perform equally skilled, yet different work. For example, the trained nurse in an intensive care unit may well be involved in monitoring and working an array of complex mechanical equipment and monitoring and responding to rapid changes in the vital signs of their patients, in order to safeguard them during the critical few hours or days following major surgery; whilst the nurse in a ward for the long-term care of elderly people finds her skills taxed in other ways, such as the feeding of a patient whose mobility is severely restricted and requires help with the most elementary human needs. Again, the Registered Mental Nurse may turn a game of cards with a very depressed client into a way of encouraging self-esteem and interaction with others and a means of assessing memory, concentration and motivation. In the past, these latter two forms of nursing skill have tended to be undervalued, both by other professionals and by nurses themselves, but the balance has, to a great extent, been redressed so that the validity of these apparently simple skills is now much more recognized within the profession.

Finally, all nurses will acquire and require competence in skills of communication and the organization of patient care, both of which require considerable application to gain, but are essential to good care.

In examining the qualities of the nurse, I have identified being caring, fit and intelligent as the three key elements. It is worth stressing that none of these qualities is inborn. If you are aware that you currently lack the formal education needed to undertake nurse training, this is not something which needs to hold you back indefinitely. Nursing courses are accustomed to dealing with people with widely differing educational backgrounds, either by offering them additional input during their training or directing them towards 'access' education which helps prepare them for nurse training. Similarly, fitness is something which we can work at; indeed in nursing we often require patients to do exactly that! Caring is not some mystical quality, but something which we learn, often very early in our lives. Learning how to *express* caring, however, is different, and in many ways nurse training involves just this.

EXERCISE

I hope you will do this exercise twice – now and when you finish reading this book. Here is a list of arguments for and against being a nurse:

For
Nursing is a job which is personally rewarding.
Nursing is about people, not things.
Nursing has exciting parts to it.
Nursing is intellectually satisfying.
Nurses are held in high esteem by society.
Nursing is almost infinitely varied.
Nursing allows you to help others.
Nursing is a comparatively secure job.

Against
Nursing is physically hard work.
Nursing is poorly paid.
Nurses are undervalued by other professions.
Nursing is emotionally draining.
Nurses work unsocial hours.
Nursing is very stressful.
Nursing takes over a part of your life.

1. Read the list carefully.
2. Spend a few minutes thinking of additions you would make to both the 'For' and 'Against' lists, and write these down.

3. Consider the lists again. This time decide how important each item on each list is to you. You might even rate each one, say on a 1 to 10 scale.
4. How do the two lists balance up for you? If you have used the scoring approach, which has the highest set of scores? Write down how confident you feel now that nursing is or is not for you.

   After you've read the book, do the exercise again. If the book has done its job, you should feel more confident about your decision, as well as having gained a good deal in the way of practical knowledge about training and working as a nurse.

Notes

1. Donne, John (1624/1975) *Devotions on Emergent Occasions*. Meditation XVII. (Edited by Anthony Raspa). Montreal: McGill-Queens University Press. (Also in many anthologies).

SECTION 2
TRAINING TO BE A NURSE

Training and education of nurses in Britain has undergone a period of unprecedented change over the past few years. Fewer nurses are being trained, but are receiving an education of far greater academic merit, whilst still seeking to retain the practical flavour for which many nurses enter the profession. Nurse educators have sought to promote the concept of the nurse as a 'knowledgeable doer' – someone who undertakes a great deal of practical work but is aware of the reasons why she undertakes this work and the theoretical elements which underpin her practice.

The two most major changes have been the achievement of student status and the shift in nurse education from a focus on illness to an emphasis on health and its promotion. Until recently, with the exception of a very small number of university students, the majority of student nurses were trained in schools of nursing. They formed a large and important part of the NHS workforce, being paid for carrying out clinical work (often with considerable responsibility) while studying for registration as a nurse alongside this work. This in turn led to a tension between the roles of student and worker and to practical difficulties in organizing study.

Today, the student role is far more central to nurse education, and nurse training is arranged according to educational rather than service needs. Colleges of nursing aim to design a programme which prepares people to be nurses in a structured way, where clinical experiences reflect and build upon educational experiences within the colleges. In the clinical areas, staff are rapidly coming to accept that student nurses are no longer to be considered merely a 'pair of hands' to help with carrying out the simpler tasks of patient care. In their turn, nursing students are expected to be more aware and questioning than ever before.

The second key change to our education of nurses has been the move towards a clear focus on the healthy individual as a core element of nurse training. Nursing has always been regarded primarily as a role involving caring for sick people, and our training has reflected this, focusing on the tasks, attitudes and knowledge required to deliver or organize such care. As a profession, nursing now sees its role as far broader than this. Certainly, nurses will always continue to care for the sick person, although the context in which that care takes place is increasingly likely to be the community as a whole, rather than the institution. However, the focus of that care will increasingly reflect what is held by many nurses to be the distinctive contribution of nursing: the ability to see and respond to individuals in their care as whole people. This implies the ability to see the health and wellness context in which the individual dwells. As part of this process of moving towards education of nurses in positive health care, all students now undergo a programme of education which begins with the well person. Since Project 2000 training was initiated, all nurses have undergone a common core of training involving a variety of theoretical and clinical subjects, all of which focus on the healthy individual. Only after 18 months, when this foundation has been completed, does the student focus in detail upon the ill person and upon the client group which she will eventually become trained to care for.

Intending students, particularly those who have prior knowledge of the work of the nurse, may find these two changes confusing, if they were expecting a training which focuses immediately on practical care of the sick. Balanced against this, the advantage to be gained from being truly a student is one for which nurse educators fought hard and long, and, it is hoped, will allow nursing students to become more thoughtful and less stressed as they progress to becoming confident and sensitive trained nurses.

In the following section, the authors set out in detail the two main ways in which it is now possible to train as a nurse: diploma- and degree-level training. Both these routes to qualification as a nurse are now based upon Project 2000 lines, and chapter 2 describes what Project 2000 means for nursing education and how it is organized. It is likely that all nurse education in the UK will eventually be to degree level, and many nurses are already seeking to upgrade their education to this level. In chapter 3, Margaret Clarke, an experienced nursing academic, describes what is distinctive about degree-level education for nurses and the role of the undergraduate nurse in both academic and clinical settings. She also outlines some of the innovative departures which have been made from the two dominant forms of pre-registration nursing education.

CHAPTER 2
Project 2000 training

Caroline Plews

WHAT IS PROJECT 2000?

If you decide to train as a professional nurse, the Project 2000
Diploma in Nursing courses will almost certainly be the first option
you examine: they are the main professional training route for
people who want to become nurses in the UK. The minimum qualification for a trained nurse is now a diploma, and this represents a
departure from previous nursing courses, which were essentially
practical certificates. The current Project 2000 courses that we will
be considering in this chapter are different from the old certificate
courses in structure, content and academic level. They are student-
focused, community- and health-orientated and academically
demanding. If you have spoken to friends and acquaintances who are
trained nurses, it is most likely that they trained under the old
certificate system, since the first nurses to undertake Project 2000
training have only just begun to qualify. So it may be helpful if we
begin by examining how the change from certificate- to diploma-
level education of nurses came into being.

Project 2000 courses are the outcome of a radical review of all
nurse education that took place in the mid-1980s,[1] carried out by the
body responsible for setting the standards for training and professional conduct of all nurses, the United Kingdom Central Council
for Nursing, Midwifery and Health Visiting (UKCC). There had
been concern for some time that the traditional method of training
had serious flaws. The main problem was that students were

contributing heavily to the workforce in the wards and other clinical areas where they were being trained. This set up a potential conflict between the needs of the student to learn and the needs of the client, who required care. Under this earlier system, for example, you might, as a student, have reached the stage where taking part in a ward round was a necessary experience to broaden your understanding and ability to work in a multidisciplinary team and to develop your professional confidence. However, if you were needed, at the same time, to deliver care to clients, then this would take precedence, and you would lose the learning opportunity. Of course, there may have been further chances for you to take part in a ward round, but such a training system was necessarily patchy in the support that it could give to learners' needs.

In addition, the status of students as members of the workforce also led to problems for organizing the clinical work. It was argued that the huge reliance on students who only stayed on the ward for two to three months led to a fragmented delivery of care; and because the students were still training, the quality of care was at times not as good as it might have been.

These issues were sharpened by the realization that the number of 18-year-olds in the population was dropping. This age group was the major source of recruitment to nursing, and it was predicted that workforce problems could arise if reliance on student labour was not reduced. Finally, it was recognized that patterns of health care were changing, rather than diminishing, and that a growing number of individuals would survive past retirement age, many of them needing a network of different types of support, including health needs.

As a result, two issues were clear. First, the falling numbers of school leavers meant that suitable potential entrants to nursing would have an increasing array of choice of education and career. Nursing education, therefore, had to become competitive with other professions, in order to attract entrants from the smaller pool. Second, it was acknowledged that future health care was going to broaden out to seek a more varied approach to health issues. Future practitioners in nursing would, therefore, require new skills, such as the ability to identify potential problems and devise health promotion strategies, and to work with all those other disciplines connected with health care issues.

The Project 2000 educational programmes of today are thus very different from the old certificate courses; society is changing quickly, and so are its professional roles and skills. Project 2000 is concerned with educating you to be a bold practitioner, who will have a knowledge of nursing within a social and political context. This will prepare you to develop your skills and intellect as the profession matures. Above all, as part of Project 2000 education, you will learn how to be an enquiring practitioner – in other words, you'll learn *how to learn*, to help you equip yourself for your continuing professional development.

Not surprisingly, the educational level of the pre-registration course is now at diploma rather than certificate level as on the traditional courses. This fits in well with the notion of progressive educational attainment. On completion of a Project 2000 course, you will find a variety of 'top-up' courses available to allow you to bring your diploma up to a degree level in nursing. Other degree courses and vocational courses will also accept either all or part of your diploma in granting exemption from some of their required study.

ORGANIZATION OF PROJECT 2000 COURSES

As a prospective student, you have the choice of qualifying in one of the four branches of nursing: adult, child, mental health and learning disabilities. More specific information about each speciality can be found in the relevant chapters in Section 3. The number of places in a particular branch is fixed according to an estimate of future staffing levels in the geographical area where you want to train. You normally need to decide which branch you wish to qualify in when you apply for a place at a college of nursing. Students do occasionally change their minds about branches during their training, but because of the fixed number of training places it will not necessarily be possible to change your speciality.

Whichever branch you choose, you'll share the first part of the course with all students who begin the course at the same time. This is because of a recognition within the profession that all branches of nursing share large common areas of certain types of knowledge and skill. Nursing has developed beyond a narrow medical model where primacy was given to knowledge of pathology and of the medical and nursing interventions required, towards a broad-based, health-centred discipline.

The first half of the programme is known as the common foundation programme and lasts 18 months, most of that time being spent in academic study, although there are also practical placements throughout. The placements may vary in nature and will not all be within institutional settings; you may find yourself working in a school, observing how such a community can help or hinder development of a healthy lifestyle. Alternatively you may be placed with a fitness centre to find out the what motivates some people to change their lifestyle. In all placements you should be given learning guidelines to help you gain the most possible benefit.

The nursing experience at this point will be in the form of placements for a few weeks on each branch area so that, by the end of the common foundation programme you will have worked briefly in all the four branches. As a student nurse, you have a very distinct status in the clinical areas because you are supernumerary, that is, you are not included in the actual workforce numbers of the particular area in which you are working. This is a radical departure from the traditional style of training where the student was also 'a pair of hands', working at least as hard on practical tasks as members of the permanent staff. Being supernumerary will give you the opportunity to develop skills and knowledge according to your own needs and not just if the ward situation will allow. However, nursing areas are complex situations where clients' needs take priority; students learn the important skills of flexibility and negotiation when working through their learning aims.

To help you get the most out of your placements you will be allocated a mentor – a registered nurse who acts as your guide and teacher in the practical area. Although most staff are very positive towards students, having a mentor means you have a nominated person whom you know has a specific role to help you get the most out of your experience. All colleges have different schedules of assessment of their students; however, all programmes will require you to reach a certain standard in both nursing and academic skills. Clinically, your mentor will have responsibility for judging whether you have reached a satisfactory level of performance for your stage in training. Academic work, usually a mixture of essays, exams and project work, is marked by college of nursing staff. It is usual to have a framework of supervision, so that you always have someone with whom to discuss a particular assignment.

The methods of teaching you experience and the size of group in which you are taught are likely to be varied. Traditionally, most schools of nursing had reasonably small intakes of students several times a year; in this situation, even formal lectures were never large, perhaps a maximum of 30 students, and there was also greater opportunity for small-group work. Project 2000 courses only run twice a year but have more students in each group, with the result that there can be numbers in excess of 60 during the common foundation programme. Once students go into their branches the numbers will obviously drop as the initial group number divides up. However, if you are going to pursue adult branch nursing your group will remain fairly large, as adult nursing accounts for most of the student nurse numbers. Large groups do not have to be a problem; it depends to a great extent on the approach adopted by both student and teacher and the facilities available to cater for these numbers. It is a good idea to ask your prospective college about these points and to have a look at the classroom and study facilities that they have.

CONTENT OF COURSES

What is it that you actually need to know in order to become a qualified nurse? The answer may surprise you! First, the '-ologies' will be much in evidence: sociology, psychology and biology. In addition, you will learn about principles of health education and health promotion, and be expected to understand elements of the research process. A basic introduction to law and ethics applied to nursing will also be covered. Last, but quite definitely not least, will be nursing theory. The content taken from these areas will be chosen on the basis of how far they help our understanding and delivery of health care. We are interested in knowledge bases that will inform our practice, rather than being of academic interest alone. This broad-based educational approach has been followed previously in universities on their degrees in nursing. It is natural that the diploma in nursing should follow the same academic trail; a nurse utilizes knowledge from a variety of sources in carrying out her job.

EXERCISE

Read the following example, and try to consider how the various elements of knowledge contribute to the patient's care: Mr Cardew is admitted to a coronary care ward after having suffered a heart attack. He is a 45-year-old married man with two children, both under 10 years of age. Mr Cardew has a demanding manual job working as a gardener for the local council, where much of his work involves felling and pruning large trees. He enjoys sport, and is an avid football supporter. When admitted to hospital, he is in pain and is both frightened about the future in terms of his medical complaint and anxious about whether he will be able to resume his work and social activities. As his illness resolves, it is this anxiety about the future which comes most to the fore.

Looking at this brief scenario, we can see that Mr Cardew is likely to rely on the nurse for administering his drugs and oxygen properly, observing his condition and liaising with other staff as necessary. In order to do this, the nurse needs knowledge of how drugs act on the body and their interactions and side-effects. She also needs to be familiar with human physiology and how it changes during illness, so that her observations of Mr Cardew have meaning for her and she can act accordingly. Taking things a step further, perhaps Mr Cardew is a patient on a ward where a new method of managing heart attacks is being investigated. In this sort of experimental situation, the nurse needs a knowledge of the ethical and legal issues involved, both so that she can safeguard the patient's rights and inform him and his family.

An understanding of psychology will be important throughout the care the nurse gives. There are psychological aspects to the perception of pain and response to medication. Later, the nurse will give Mr Cardew the chance to voice his fears and anxieties, using knowledge derived from the psychology of human anxiety and of communication to help him express himself and search for solutions.

As a final aspect of this short scenario, nursing knowledge of sociology will inform the advice given to Mr Cardew for his recovery. Dietary and exercise information will be particularly important, and the nurse will be aware of the problems of compliance with such information associated with her patient's class and occupational group, and will tailor her advice in a way which makes it most likely he will attempt to go along with her suggestions. For example, she will suggest changes to diet which, although they are more healthy, are also as close as possible to the sort of food Mr Cardew has been used to eating.

What I want to give you is some flavour of the complexity of the nursing role as it is has developed and is developing today. The diversity of knowledge that is needed by nurses is potentially both exciting and interesting. In some cases, students enrolling on a

Project 2000 course have been daunted and disappointed when they have recognized the range of academic subjects that they are required to study. Rest assured that this academic framework is there not only to allow you to develop to your professional potential but also because adequate care of patients requires a more sophisticated knowledge base within the profession. Of course, acquiring knowledge does not necessarily make you a more caring person, but it should make you more effective in actually delivering that care.

Having discussed the type of content you can expect, it is worth examining the kind of qualities you will need to be a successful student. As in all higher education courses, there will be an emphasis on self-directed learning; that is, you can expect to have to seek out information for yourself from books and other sources, with guidelines being given to help you. Ultimately, however, it will be up to you to have the discipline and tenacity to carry out this part of your learning. This approach has two major benefits. The first is that it can give you considerable flexibility as to when you study. If you want to hit the books at 11 p.m. when there are no distractions around, there is nothing to stop you. Secondly, the self-directed approach gives you control over your own learning. This process of discovering information for yourself encourages self-reliance and confidence in studying. These are essential qualities to have as a qualified nurse when you will be responsible for your professional updating of knowledge and skills.

The idea of students being actively involved in designing and initiating their learning will also be followed on practice placements. For example, you may be placed with a district nurse mentor for a number of weeks. Although the mentor is there to support you, she should not spoonfeed you. She will be looking for a student who will be actively seeking information and asking questions about, for example, the clients they visit, how district nurse resources are allocated in that locality, the benefits and problems of care of a dying patient in the community as opposed to the hospital. Opportunities on placements can vary because of staff shortages, personality differences and the type of client contact available. However, all these variables can be lessened in impact if the student is prepared to identify any difficulties and then think of ways around them.

The majority of practical experience comes in the second 18 months of training. At this stage you have entered the branch in which you will be specializing. At intervals you will come back into college for theoretical input. Of course, academic assessments such as essays and exams continue during this time. During your final year of training, you will change your status in the training area: instead of being supernumerary you will go on what is termed rostered service. This simply means that at this point the health authority where you are receiving your training start to pay a proportion of the cost of your training. So, instead of being additional to the staff on a client area you are counted in as one of the working team. As a result, you can expect to work some evening and weekend shifts and also bank holidays. However, students are not entitled to extra money payments for weekends and bank holidays until they are qualified.

CONCLUSION

It may be tempting to see the day you pick up your diploma as the day that you say goodbye to studying. However, once qualified you will find that you need, and will be expected, to keep up to date with developments in nursing and health care. The Project 2000 course can equip you to be a confident and self directed learner. This will be important not only for the duration of your initial training course but for the rest of your career in nursing. You will be eligible to apply for entry to degree programmes as well as a huge variety of professional courses. Consequently, a decision to undertake a diploma in nursing course includes a lasting commitment to educational and professional development. Although this can sound daunting it can also mean entrance to a career path that is both challenging and interesting.

EXERCISE

1. Our discussion of Mr Cardew, his care and the knowledge required to provide it left some areas of his life uncovered. Expand on the picture given of him to consider ways in which his life might be affected. For example, might he be frightened by playing energetically with his children, or by having sex? Might he be worried about having to stop work? Make a list of these potential effects of illness on his life. Now make a note next to each item on the list of the kind of knowledge area the nurse will need in order to help him with these concerns. Naturally, you should not expect

to have that knowledge yourself, since these are the things you will learn about as a student nurse. However, doing this exercise should give you a further idea of the importance of different areas of knowledge and also introduce you to the kind of process nurses undergo when considering how to help their patients.

2. Consider whether a course at diploma level is right for you at the moment. Examine in particular whether the level is likely to be too high or too low for you. If you consider it to be too high, you should seek advice about further education before entry into Project 2000. You should also read chapter 13, which examines entry requirements in detail. If you feel the level is too low, now is a good time to turn to chapter 3, which deals with university undergraduate courses in nursing.

Notes

1. United Kingdom Central Council for Nursing, Midwifery and Health Visiting (1986) *Project 2000: A new preparation for practice*. London: UKCC.

CHAPTER 3
Undergraduate training and experimental courses

Margaret Clarke

INTRODUCTION

What do we mean when we talk about degree courses in nursing? The answer is not as obvious as it might seem, but basically we mean a course which enables an individual to study nursing up to the level at which they can be examined for the award of a degree. Usually, by such a term, we mean an undergraduate or first degree. In the case of nursing this may be a BSc, BSocSci, BA, or BNurs. Such courses usually incorporate enough clinical experience to enable the successful graduate to register as a nurse on the completion of the course.

However not all undergraduate-level courses in nursing are designed for the new entrant to the profession. Instead, one or two full-time courses and many part-time ones are designed for nurses who are already registered. Effectively they allow nurses who are not graduates to become so. It will be obvious that even with exemptions from part of the course, which may or may not be available, this way of becoming a nurse and a graduate is time consuming. Quite a number of taught masters degrees in nursing are designed in the same way, and allow non-graduate nurses to graduate. Other taught masters courses, however, are more like masters degrees in other academic subjects, and are specialist degrees to allow those who have a bachelor's degree to develop depth of knowledge in a fairly narrow subject area. Examples in nursing are masters degrees in oncology nursing, the care of elderly people or critical care nursing. In addition, it is possible to undertake research degrees in nursing, either the Master of Philosophy or a doctorate (PhD or DPhil). Added to this complexity is the fact that specialization is also possible to some extent at undergraduate level and so you can, for example, take a degree in mental health nursing.

Trained nurses can and do undertake degrees in subjects other than nursing, as many of the older lecturers in nursing at universities have done; there were once no degrees in nursing for them to take! For the rest of this chapter we are going to consider undergraduate courses for the new entrant to the nursing profession.

WHY ARE THERE DEGREE COURSES AS WELL AS DIPLOMA COURSES IN NURSING?

Many people, even today, are surprised that there are degree courses in nursing in this country. Yet the first such course, offered at the University of Edinburgh, has been in existence for almost 40 years. However it was not until 12 years later that an existing diploma course in nursing at the University of Manchester converted into a degree course and thus became the first nursing degree course in England. Following that, a number of higher education institutions established nursing departments and nursing degree courses during the next decade. An explanation of this development will help in understanding today's nursing scene.

Whilst university education has been available in the USA for some nurses during most of the current century, until that pioneering course in Edinburgh nurse training in the UK was very much an apprenticeship. It occurred mainly in the wards, and was based on the view that nursing was a vocational occupation concerned with helping the doctor to treat the sick. So-called student nurses were part of the ward workforce and so were subject to long shifts and night work. Lectures were provided at first by doctors on the ward and later in schools of nursing when students were withdrawn from the wards for 'blocks' of between two and twelve weeks at a time for study. In such a climate, where nurses were seen as needing to learn *how to do things* to a far greater extent than the theory behind the things they did, the wonder is that there was someone far-sighted enough to see the need for university education for nurses at all.

One contributing factor was a general expansion of university and polytechnic places within the UK, enabling more women to take up degree places than previously. There was a fear amongst nursing leaders that the brightest women would be 'creamed off' by the universities leaving the less educationally able to go into nursing. At the same time higher education institutions needed to fill the newly acquired places and saw that one way of attracting students was to offer a wider variety of subjects at degree level by expanding into new areas. Nursing was one of these new subject areas. Already there were forces within the nursing profession who saw the need for autonomous nursing practice and practitioners who could speak up for nursing on equal terms with other professions within the NHS. To prepare nurses by means of undergraduate programmes would, it was thought, give them the confidence in discussion enjoyed by graduate professions, in particular medicine.

Thus there was a movement toward the professionalization of nursing and the universities and polytechnics were seen as having a part to play in this. An important aspect of a profession is that its practitioners engage in research into their practice. Although there had been a little research into nursing in this country since 1956, that research was sparse and tended to be concerned with management of nursing or nursing education rather than clinical nursing. The place where research training is traditionally carried out in this country is in the universities. So here we have another reason why the setting up of departments of nursing was encouraged. University lecturers are expected to carry out research as part of their job, and research carries at least as much weight as teaching skill in consideration for promotion. By offering degree courses in nursing there would eventually be graduates to undertake research training and so increase the amount of research available.

ACADEMIC CREDIBILITY OF CONTENT OF UNDER-GRADUATE COURSES

The universities were allowed considerable freedom in designing experimental nursing courses. One of the interesting outcomes of the movement into universities and the relative freedom to devise the curriculum, was an increasing awareness of the number of subject areas in addition to nursing which are relevant to the practice of nursing. A fear, on the part of traditional academics, that nursing would become a second-class subject with no academic credibility was proved to be unjustified. Far from it being difficult to find enough subject areas to study to justify the award of a degree, those of us planning degree courses had to make conscious choices about which subjects mattered most and which could be left out. As a result, different decisions were made in different nursing departments, resulting in degree programmes which differed from one another. Some were heavily scientific, for example the degrees offered by the University of Surrey and the University of Glasgow. Others were more heavily social science based, for example the degree at the University of Edinburgh. Yet other departments balanced science and social science elements evenly. These differences, many of which persist today, had implications for the type of A-level which qualified prospective candidates for entry into the courses.

From what I have said about degree courses in nursing, I hope you can see that, in spite of some of the controversy and lack of understanding associated with development in the early days, they were successful. A striking feature of these courses was how successful they were in reducing the wastage which was a considerable problem with the more conventional certificate courses. Not only did a higher proportion of students complete the degree courses successfully, but after graduation a higher percentage stayed in nursing, particularly in patient care.[1, 2] The success of the degree courses heavily influenced the Project 2000 proposals.[3]

Given that the Project 2000 proposals were based on degree courses, clearly the difference between the diploma and undergraduate methods of studying to be a nurse has narrowed. The advantages and disadvantages of reading for a degree in nursing today are discussed in the next section.

ADVANTAGES OF AN UNDERGRADUATE COURSE IN NURSING AS A PREPARATION FOR A NURSING CAREER

One of the major benefits of going to university is the opportunity to participate in university life. It is worth noting that, nowadays, Project 2000 courses are run in association with a university and, in consequence, some of the students on such courses may have access to some or all of the social and academic facilities of the university. However, most such courses are run at a distance from the main university site and so participation is more difficult than for the students based at the university itself.

University life is both academic and social, and the social aspects are discussed in chapter 14. Apart from these social aspects of university life there is also the advantage that the subjects studied other than nursing will be taught by the subject specialists from the relevant departments. For example psychology will be taught by experts in psychology, who will be engaged in research in their subjects. Frequently, nursing students will share lectures with students undertaking honours degrees in the subject in question. Occasionally students who entered university to read nursing find that they like one of these other subjects so much that they change course. The reverse also happens when a student who embarked on a subject other than nursing decides to change to nursing. Such changes are relatively easy, especially during the first year. Another opportunity which is readily available is the series of public lectures which universities put on and the inaugural lectures, many in subjects which enhance nursing studies but also others which, although nothing to do with health care, are stimulating and broadening in their own right.

INTELLECTUAL FREEDOM AND STIMULATION

It is apparent that taking a degree in any subject is intellectually stimulating. Nursing is particularly so, since it includes many relevant subjects other than nursing. As far as the subject itself is concerned, the staff employed in the university department of nursing have a commitment to carry out research as part of their contract of employment. This means that students are being taught by people who are actively engaged in developing the knowledge base of nursing. There will be research students in the department who may give tutorials or carry out other informal teaching. Lectures may be arranged from the 'big names' in nursing.

There is now less freedom for university nursing departments to design their courses for new entrants to the profession exactly as they please and they have to conform with the guidelines laid down by the statutory bodies for Project 2000 courses. Nonetheless, it is possible for the university lecturers to include the latest knowledge, from their own research and that of their colleagues, in their teaching. Many staff act as consultants to clinical staff, government bodies, health authorities and NHS trusts, whilst others carry out editorial work for the learned nursing journals. Although this may mean that they are not always readily available within their departments, it does result in their bringing a breadth of vision about nursing to their teaching. For the university student, this leads to the stimulation of being in contact with teachers who are genuinely at the forefront of expanding nursing knowledge.

Whilst all nursing courses now include research appreciation, the degree courses usually devote more hours to this subject. Most degree courses include an opportunity for an individual research project to be carried out by the undergraduate, usually in the final year. This is an excellent opportunity for students to experience what it is like to do research, and to discover whether or not they wish to take it further by undertaking a research degree or pursuing a career in research. In general, the size of the cohorts of students taking degree courses is smaller than for the comparable Project 2000 course, so there may be more individual attention available from teaching staff. Unfortunately, financial considerations mean the universities have to be cost effective and this has tended to mean that class sizes have increased. There is no doubt, however, that the relationships between university teachers and students are informal and personal. Staff get to know individual students partly through the personal tutorial system, whereby each member of academic staff is responsible for the pastoral care of a number of students.

One of the strong characteristics of university life is that responsibility for learning is placed firmly on the students themselves. Lecture attendance is not policed in any way, although students may be required to attend tutorials, seminars and practical work. Students are expected, however, to learn the work covered in lectures and to use what they have learned in assessed work and examinations. Seminar work at university level is particularly valuable in learning to present one's work for critical discussion by others, learning to be objective about it and learning the skills of defending one's own work intellectually. This gives confidence which is extremely useful when, as a trained nurse, you are asked to teach patients and other nurses.

In general, although subject to the rules of the nursing statutory body, it does seem easier for university students to take time out from their studies for such activities as membership of national sports teams, voluntary work or becoming an official of the students' union.

These then are some of the advantages of taking a nursing degree course at university. There are, of course, disadvantages as well, and I shall now discuss these.

DISADVANTAGES OF BEING AN UNDERGRADUATE

There is no doubt that all students at university are feeling financial hardship. However, nursing students may have additional demands on their finance since they have to engage in clinical work as part of the requirement for registration as a nurse; and clinical work inevitably means travel. Even if the nursing department is situated in a medical school within a hospital, quite a lot of clinical experience must be gained away from hospitals and in the community. This means the students must travel to doctors' surgeries, health centres and patients' homes, for example. An element of the grant is for travel and students can claim from their local education authority, for travel which is essential to their course, over and above this amount. Unfortunately, however, such claims can only be made at the end of the term during which the student has incurred the expenditure, so the student has to pay for the travel before receiving the reimbursement. In contrast, Project 2000 students not only receive a non-means tested bursary but also have their travel expenses paid.

Whilst it is not easy for any student to obtain employment during vacations, this is virtually impossible for nursing students, since their degree courses operate during vacation time as well as during the normal term times, so that there is little opportunity available for paid employment. Nursing students need to buy books, calculators and so on, like any other student. In addition it may be necessary to buy uniform at the start of the course, since, like everyone else these days, the NHS Trusts are cutting costs and the provision of uniform has stopped, even in those places where it used to be provided.

NURSING DEGREES AND OTHER UNDERGRADUATE COURSES

So far, I have been comparing nursing degree courses, either implicitly or explicitly, with the Project 2000 diploma courses. Perhaps it is time to compare them with degree courses in other subjects. There is no doubt that in comparison with other subjects nursing is very challenging and can be stressful. This is partly because of the breadth of the subject matter studied, but the clinical work is also a major factor. During clinical experience the student moves gradually from being mainly an observer, responsible only for such activities as could be done by a lay person, to taking on more and more responsibility. The aim is to prepare the student to become a fully professional trained nurse and this cannot be done without preparation for the responsibility to come. As well as responsibility toward the end of the course, there is the emotional investment made throughout it. Inevitably one does get involved with the lives of the patients and clients one sees, and cares about the outcomes of health care for them; this takes its emotional toll. It is one reason why it is so useful to know that universities have professional counsellors on hand, as well as nursing lecturers who understand, having been nurses themselves. It is also fair to say that such emotional investment is very rewarding. Indeed one of the comments I have heard academics from other subjects say about nursing students is how mature and socially skilled they are compared with the average undergraduate. Another complimentary comment that has been made many times is about the academic ability of nursing students and their commitment to the subject.

A clear difference between most degree courses and nursing degrees is that the majority of undergraduate nursing courses for new entrants to the profession are four years in length rather than three; this is also a telling point of difference compared with the Project 2000 courses. In practical terms it means that the graduate is looking for employment a year later than a Project 2000 student who started to study at the same time. There will be no financial advantage to the graduate, either, who will usually start work, in the NHS at least, on the same salary as a diplomate nurse. The graduate may make up for this disadvantage later in improved employment and promotion prospects, but this is by no means certain. However, there is a strong possibility that nursing will become an all-graduate profession in the future; when this happens, the graduate nurse will have a clear advantage. Similarly, even today, many nurses are rushing to 'top-up' their certificates and diplomas on conversion degree courses, often because they require the degree in order to compete for higher grades in the hospitals and other settings where they work. This is particularly difficult because they are, by the time they seek such promotion, mature people, often with family commitments.

Once again, the nurse whose basic education is to degree level may gain, because she does not have either to take a career break or study part-time later on in order to upgrade her qualification. As a sign that the degree will become essential, it should be noted that it is now virtually a requirement if one wishes to teach nurses or undertake research. The degree nurse has the advantage, therefore, of potentially greater flexibility of career earlier. As one example, I recently employed a graduate nurse, in a research capacity, who had done no clinical nursing at all, other than her training, and who wanted to pursue a career in nursing research quite separate from clinical involvement. This would have been an impossible choice in nursing ten years ago, and remains so for the non-graduate nurse.

DEGREES IN MIDWIFERY AND OTHER NURSING COURSES

I have mentioned above that the university departments no longer have the amount of freedom to offer their own theoretical curriculum that they once enjoyed. This is because in accepting the Project 2000 recommendations the government had to set up new statutory bodies. As a part of this, the legislation covering nurse training is now different and all courses of basic nursing preparation have to conform to Project 2000 principles. However it is only fair to say that all course teams now have a reasonable amount of freedom to plan a course which suits local circumstances, provided that it conforms in broad outline to the recommendations of the National Boards.

This has had consequences for the university departments of nursing, which until recently usually offered a degree in only one type of nursing for new entrants to the profession, which in the vast majority of cases was adult general nursing. With the implementation of the Project 2000 recommendations, all institutions offering courses of preparation to new entrants to the profession were asked to offer four branch programmes. These were the courses that led to qualifications in adult nursing, children's nursing, mental health nursing or nursing of people with a learning disability.

Since the original ruling it has been realized that university departments do not have the resources available to offer four courses of this kind; this was particularly so where specialist staff were concerned. Therefore the policy has been changed and whilst there is encouragement to offer two branch programmes leading to degrees, it is possible to make out a case for running only one branch. This has meant that different university departments of nursing offer anything from one to four degrees leading to qualifications on different parts of the Nursing Register held at the UKCC.

Midwifery courses are treated differently from nursing courses. Whilst all courses leading to a qualification allowing the individual to practise as a midwife must be at least at higher education diploma level, it is common to take a midwifery course after qualification as a nurse; however it is possible to take a course of direct entry to midwifery without being a nurse first. This has led to just one or two centres offering undergraduate courses in midwifery which are

designed for new entrants to the profession. Most of the considerations which apply to nursing degree courses also apply to midwifery
courses. However the staff running such courses will be midwives
and will be engaged in carrying out research into midwifery as well
as teaching undergraduate student midwives.

DEGREES IN NURSING AND MIDWIFERY AND THE NURSING PROFESSION

My comments above about the importance of degree courses and
academic departments of nursing and midwifery for the professionalization of these professions remain true today. Perhaps it is even
more important now that there is a new grade of health care assistant
working in the NHS. This has meant rethinking what particular
benefits are brought to patient care by highly trained nurses.
Another development in progress is the reduction of junior doctors'
working hours in hospital, with many nurses taking on some of the
duties previously carried out by junior doctors. This has great benefits to patients, who receive holistic care from a nurse who knows
them well, rather than having some procedures carried out by a
doctor who does not know them and who, due to tiredness, is not at
the peak of alertness .

Nursing and midwifery are changing to meet the changing health
care needs of society. There is no doubt that the university departments are playing a large part in the research and teaching which has
to underpin these changes. Graduates in nursing and midwifery play
a particularly crucial role in this, having had a preparation which
enables them not only to cope well with change but to help in
shaping that change.

EXERCISE

1. List reasons why you believe university education for
    nurses is important for the nursing profession. Beside
    each of the reasons you have listed, write brief notes about
    why this reason is important to you. For instance, perhaps
    you want a deeper level of study of biology than a diploma
    will provide. This is a clear *current* reason for choosing a
    degree course. By contrast, you may already firmly want a

career within the university system, doing teaching and research. If you have decided this, it is a reason concerning your *future* for undertaking a degree now.

2. Spend a couple of minutes considering what kind of person you are, and then identify the advantages and disadvantages of an undergraduate course in nursing or midwifery *for you*. Write out a list of these for yourself. How important are the disadvantages? Can you think of ways you will cope with them in order to achieve your aim?

Notes

1. Kemp, J. (1988) 'Graduates in nursing: a report of a longitudinal study at the University of Hull'. *Journal of Advanced Nursing 13*, 281–7.
2. Marsh, N. (1976) 'Summary report of a study on the career paths of diplomates/graduates of the undergraduate nursing course in the University of Manchester.' *Journal of Advanced Nursing 1*, 539–62.
3. United Kingdom Central Council for Nursing, Midwifery and Health Visiting (1986) *Project 2000: A new preparation for practice*. London, UKCC.

SECTION 3
WORKING AS A NURSE

From your reading of the previous section, you will now have a fair idea of how today's nurses are educated. One thing which emerges clearly is the complexity of what we now do as nurses. The education we undertake mirrors this complexity, but cannot fully equip us for our role as experts in human health care. Project 2000 is a great advance in nursing education because it is such a broad preparation for practice, and because the picture it gives us of the human being in health and illness is likewise broad. Furthermore, both students and teachers are more able to concentrate on educational aspects of nurse training, since these have finally been decoupled from the need for student nurses to provide a service. As a result, we can expect the first nursing diplomates to have been much better educated than their counterparts on traditional courses.

However, it is now generally accepted that these new diplomates will have much still to learn in the clinical setting, once they have qualified and are faced with the need to form part of a service-led workforce, with the differing demands this will make upon them. Fortunately, nurse educators and service providers are coming to recognize that it is no longer sufficient to expect the newly qualified staff nurse simply to carry on from where she left off as a student, and are recognizing that the early months of practice are a consolidation period during which the nurse comes to grips with a great many issues as she continues to learn. Indeed, formal periods of induction and 'preceptorship', in which an experienced nurse works with her newly qualified counterpart to explore issues related to developing as a clinical practitioner, are becoming a much more prominent feature of the life of the recently qualified nurse. This illustrates that it has now been recognized that early practice as a qualified nurse is a key time for the clinician.

We cannot, when first deciding on a career in nursing, be aware of where our choices will lead us. Many of these decisions can only truly be made when we start to have some idea about what it really means to work as a nurse, accountable for our actions and responsible on a minute-by-minute basis for our interventions with clients and patients. Yet it is usually the case that student nurses are required to decide at the beginning of their training which clinical pathway they will follow for the next three years. Sometimes an element of flexibility is allowable in choosing between the branch programmes at later points in the common foundation programme, but this is comparatively rare.

The beginning nurse is, therefore, in the position of having to attempt to gain some kind of idea about how practising nurses function in their clinical roles when caring for the adult, the child, the person with mental health problems and the person with learning disabilities. Each of these categories represents a separate route which must be chosen, almost always before education is commenced, and certainly within the first 18 months of training. The roles and duties associated with the four branch programmes are widely different, often requiring different skills, areas of knowledge and, quite possibly, different personal attributes and attitudes. You may, as an intending nurse, have embarked upon training with a strong desire to care for one particular group of people. Whilst this is, in itself, quite excellent, and potentially takes all the difficulty out of deciding between the branches, there are two possible issues. The first is a general one: your impressions of what is required of you by a particular branch of nursing may not, in fact, match the reality of working as a nurse in that field. The second is more specific: a great many people, when they first consider nursing, are simply unaware of the different forms of nursing training available. Where this is the case, people most often assume that adult nursing is the only nurse training, or is a prerequisite for the other forms of training. At the very least, since nurses who care for adults are by far the most numerous group in nursing, it is most likely that intending nurses will have come into contact with them. As a result, the most readily available source of first-hand knowledge of working as a nurse relates to nursing the adult.

Which of the major elements of nursing will you eventually want to pursue, after the initial 18 months of the common foundation programme, and how do nurses fair during the early stages of their work following training? In this section, we try to show you how nurse education translates into clinical work by creating a series of realistic pictures of the four main areas of nursing (adults, children, mental health and learning disabilities), as likely to be experienced by nurses in the early months or years following qualification. In particular, we hope you will, as a result of reading these chapters, emerge with a clear idea of the kinds of clinical and other issues nurses working in these areas come into contact with, and the skills required of them in facing these issues.

All the chapters follow a similar general approach, giving you examples from the working lives of nurses and drawing general principles from these examples. By the end of the section, you should have a fair idea of what to expect after qualifying as a nurse in each of the four areas covered.

CHAPTER 4
Nursing adults

Peter Draper

INTRODUCTION

Many people, if asked to think of a nurse, would conjure up an image of a woman, dressed in a traditional uniform, working at the bedside of patients in hospital. Certain aspects of this picture are quite reasonable: adult nursing is the biggest branch of the nursing profession, and many adult nurses work in hospital settings in the traditional way. However, my purpose in this chapter is to show you that the modern profession of adult nursing is a good deal more complex, interesting and varied than this picture allows. Adult nurses work in hospitals, schools, hospices, industrial settings, in the community and in many other places. Their roles encompass an enormous range of different functions: educating the healthy, caring for the sick, giving advice to employers about the health needs of their staff, prescribing certain drugs in community health centres, teaching children about sexual health, conducting research, and managing hospitals.

Despite this enormous range of functions, there are a number of common features to most of the jobs that adult nurses do, and we will open the chapter by examining some of these. As the chapter develops, we will take look at the job profiles of two different adult nurses: Nicky Jackson, who is a primary nurse in a rehabilitation ward for older people, and Mike Harris, an associate nurse responsible for the care of adults with blood disorders such as leukaemia.

CONTACT WITH PATIENTS AND CLIENTS

The most obvious thing that all adult nurses have in common is their involvement in the 'care' of other adults. I have put the word 'care' in inverted commas here because I want to be specific about its meaning. The word 'care' can sometimes suggest a process of looking after someone who is rather passive and helpless, such as a small baby, who cannot 'care' for himself, and will therefore need skilled help for the foreseeable future; it is quite unusual for nursing care to be of this type. Most of the people for whom nurses care have very specific problems and can eventually look forward to an independent future. The nurse's job is to offer support while it is needed, and give people the skill, strength or knowledge that will help them to be self-reliant. Spend a few moments on the exercise given at the end of the chapter; it will encourage you to consider the types of health-related problems that people experience, and the kind of help they need as a consequence. In the following example, we see a nurse carrying out a series of apparently simple interactions with clients which, in fact, require sensitivity and skill.

CASE STUDY

Professional profile: Nicky Jackson
Nicky Jackson is primary nurse in a rehabilitation ward for older people. She has been a Registered Nurse for two years, her qualifications being RN (Registered Nurse) and DipHE (Diploma in Higher Education), which she gained at her local college of nursing and midwifery. She is on the 'E' grade of the salary scale, which means that she is a senior staff nurse. As such, she is expected to work in a relatively autonomous way, and is responsible for supervising the work of less experienced colleagues

As a primary nurse, Nicky is responsible for every aspect of the nursing care of a group of eight elderly patients on the ward on which she works. This does not mean that she personally has to deliver that care – she directs the work of a team of less experienced associate nurses, who assist her in care delivery – but that she is accountable for it. In other words, she has to ensure that the care is appropriate to the needs of her patients, and is of good quality.

Today, Nicky's patients range in age from 69 to 84 and are suffering from a variety of nursing and medical problems. For example, Mrs Simpson has heart failure, which causes her legs to swell and makes it difficult for her to exert herself; Mr Armstrong has recently had a rather severe stroke, which has left him unable to speak coherently, and made him very dependent on the nursing staff; and Mr Reece, who has Parkinson's disease, is in for his regular two-week period of respite care, so that the daughter who normally cares for him at home can have a break.

Nicky begins her day by reading through notes made by the night staff about the progress of the patients, and by reviewing the care that they have received. Next she visits each of the patients with the associate nurse who will be working with that patient, taking the care plan along with her; the purpose of this visit is to discuss the day's care with the patient and the associate nurse. Nicky knows from nursing research that most patients prefer to be involved in decisions about their care. Although she is unable to hold a conversation with Mr Armstrong, she sits by him on the bed and holds his hand whilst describing to him the care that he will receive during the morning. She is unable to tell whether or not he understands.

From this point onwards, most of Nicky's day is spent in direct patient care. She helps to bath Mr Armstrong and, in consultation with the ward physiotherapist, places him in the position that will help to promote his recovery. Later in the day she will ring Mr Armstrong's wife to discuss the progress that he is making. During the day, most of Nicky's time is occupied by practical activities such as supervizing patients as they dress, encouraging people to walk, administering medications, and arranging social functions that also have a therapeutic purpose.

In the late morning, Nicky is involved in the multidisciplinary case conference, in which nurses, medical staff, therapists and any other relevant professionals discuss the progress that patients have made, and make arrangements for continuing care or discharge.

After lunch, Nicky is involved in a formal audit of the quality of care on the ward adjoining her own. The audit involves scrutinizing documentation, talking to nursing staff, and most importantly, talking to patients. In a few days, the care provided to her own patients will be audited by a visiting nurse, in a similar way.

Nicky's immediate career goal is to undertake a degree in nursing studies at her local university, but in order to get the degree she will need to study for two years, part time. This will be difficult, because her employer will not provide assistance with fees, and she will have to attend the university on one of her weekly days off. However, she knows that the degree qualification will be to the ultimate benefit of her career

NURSING ROLES

Anyone who is thinking of becoming a general nurse ought to spend some time thinking about the kinds of things that nurses do as they care for others, and about the implications of offering physical care to another adult human being. As we see in Nicky's profile, nurses often do the things which people normally do for themselves within their own homes: dressing, washing, eating, drinking, and so on. A senior colleague once said to me that 'Nursing is what people's mothers do.' She did not mean by this that the job of nursing is uniquely suitable for women (although some feminist historians of nursing point out that nursing is heir to an ancient tradition of healing as women's work), but that nursing is a 'nurturing' profession. Indeed, the words 'nurse' and 'nourish' are both drawn from the same root. However, one important difference between nursing in the home and professional nursing is that the latter activity involves working with strangers. We will now discuss the implications of this fact.

Every human society has an unwritten system of rules or 'norms' which regulate day-to-day behaviour. We learn these norms as children, during the process of being brought up or 'socialized'. It is very unusual to think about these rules, and you would probably find it rather difficult to put them all in a list, but they do exist, and they exert a very powerful regulating effect on our behaviour. We often only think about the effect of these rules if we find ourselves in a situation in which a different set of rules applies, for example when we go on holiday to a country with a different culture.

The process of giving physical care to another person often involves situations in which the normal rules of interpersonal conduct are suspended. Under certain circumstances, society gives nurses the licence to see people who are unclothed, to touch parts of their bodies or bodily products, and to cause pain. Eventually, nurses become accustomed to 'breaking the rules' in this way, as they learn that the nurse–patient relationship is regulated by a different set of norms; but the newcomer to nursing may find herself confronted by powerful feelings and emotions such as revulsion, embarrassment, grief, or sexual attraction. In the initial stages of her career, the nurse may find that these powerful feelings are very difficult to cope with. There is, of course, the opposite danger that the experienced nurse becomes blasé and unmoved, and is no longer able to empathize with the patient's experience.

These issues are only a part of the nursing role. Adult nurses are also involved, in varying degrees, in a range of functions that are extremely dissimilar to anything that occurs in people's homes. Many of these functions require special knowledge and skills, which are often learned on post-registration courses. For instance, nurses who work in intensive care units are skilled in the care of people whose breathing is assisted by mechanical ventilators, whilst those who work in renal units set up and operate dialysis machines (artificial kidneys). Many ward-based nurses also have special technical skills. It would be a mistake to think that nurses who work in 'high-tech' areas are necessarily more skilled than those who work, for instance, with older people in an ordinary ward. Contrary to expectation, research has shown that nurses whose work involves them most closely with doctors tend to take fewer decisions and are less autonomous in their practice. In other words, it does not automatically follow that nurses who possess a high degree of technical skill or manual dexterity carry more responsibility than their colleagues in other fields.

COMMUNICATION

Communication is a central aspect of the work of all nurses, as important in adult nursing as in any other branch. Some aspects of the nurse's role as communicator are quite obvious, as in teaching, for example. Very often, patients and clients need to learn new skills. Consider, for example, the case of the person who develops diabetes. In order to live independently, diabetics need to learn how to measure the amount of sugar in their urine and blood, and then to inject the correct amount of insulin. Adult nurses – sometimes in hospital but more often in the community – play an important role in teaching these new skills, and their success in doing this depends upon their skill as communicators. Similarly, nurses need communication skills of a high order when they are breaking bad news to patients or bereaved relatives. In these circumstances, it is important to choose clear and simple words whose meaning cannot be misunderstood, to provide written information for the person to refer to later if this is appropriate, and to be a skilful listener. Every nurse's education equips her with the communication skills that are needed in situations such as these.

Other aspects of the nurse's role as a communicator are not quite so obvious. An enormous amount of information is generated about hospital patients, some of which is written or printed on paper, and goes to make up the formal medical and nursing notes. These notes must be carefully maintained, as they provide a record of the patient's current status and decisions that have been made about their treatment. Increasingly, this information is stored on computer, calling for nurses to learn new skills in data management. However, a lot of the information with which nurses are concerned does not exist in written form. Nurses are constantly involved in patient assessment and monitoring the effectiveness of the care that has been given. This information must then be communicated to other nurses, to colleagues such as physiotherapists and doctors, and, of course, back to the patients themselves. This occurs during day-to-day work, and also during semi-formal meetings such as case conferences and ward rounds. The management of information is one of the most important aspects of the role of the adult nurse. Mike Harris, in the example which follows, shows us how conflicts relating to information transmission can create challenges during care.

CASE STUDY

Professional profile: Mike Harris

Mike Harris is newly qualified as a Registered Nurse who trained while studying as an undergraduate in nursing at his local university; consequently he now holds the degree of BSc (Hons) Nursing as well as the RN qualification. Following graduation, Mike hoped that he would be able to get a job on the surgical unit of his local district general hospital. Unfortunately, there were many more applicants than vacancies, but he feels lucky to have got a job on the haematology ward, and is pleased to find that the work is intellectually challenging as well as being professionally rewarding. Mike is paid at the 'D' grade, and his formal job title is that of associate nurse. Staff nurses at 'D' grade usually lack experience, and normally work under the supervision of a more senior colleague often designated as a primary nurse.

Mike's patients are aged between 18 and 65. Medically they suffer from a range of diseases, including anaemia, AIDS, and several different forms of leukaemia. These diseases impact upon every part of the lives of his patients and their relatives, and Mike finds that his job extends well beyond physical care, to include a counselling and advisory component that draws upon all the interpersonal and communication skills that he developed as an undergraduate.

Today, Mike has to find a way of balancing the conflicting demands of two parts of his job. His position as an associate nurse means that he is responsible for the physical care of a group a patients, and he wants to be ready for a case conference with the senior consultant at 2.00 p.m. However, he is also aware that the parents of one of his patients, a boy in his early teens, are trying to come to terms with the implications of a diagnosis of leukaemia. It is unlikely that the disease will be fatal, but its treatment will require frequent periods of treatment in hospital, and this will impose a severe financial burden upon the family.

Mike's way of solving this dilemma is to spend most of his time with the leukaemic boy and his family; consequently, he is ill-prepared for the case conference, and feels guilty for not leaving the ward as tidy as he knows the ward manager likes it to be. As Mike prepares to go home at the end of the day, he feels dissatisfied with what he has managed to achieve. He talks briefly with his primary nurse, who gives him credit for spending most of his time on an invisible but important priority, and assures him that ward tidiness is of secondary importance. She promises to discuss priority setting and time management with him when she gets the opportunity.

PLANNING AND ORGANIZATION

Adult nurses are involved in planning and organizing both the care of individual patients, and the systems of care which operate in various wards and departments. The care of individual patients is normally based on a problem-solving approach called the 'nursing process', which normally consists of five stages. During the *assessment* stage, the nurse interviews the person, and may perform a physical examination, in order to understand the way in which their normal state of health has been compromized. This leads to the statement of a number of *problems*, or *nursing diagnoses*. The third stage is one of *planning*, during which the nurse, in consultation with the patient, establishes the goals of treatment and considers the resources that are available before deciding treatment priorities and setting likely outcomes. During the stage of *intervention*, the nurse executes the treatment plan. This may, for example, involve dressing a wound in a particular way, or implementing a programme of exercise for the patient recovering from a heart attack. The final stage is one of *evaluation*, where the nurse reviews the outcome of treatment before beginning the cycle again with a repeated assessment, if this appears to be necessary.

As well as planning the care of individual patients, nurses are also responsible for planning the care of groups of patients. In the hospital setting, this commonly is done according to the *primary nursing* approach, which has replaced a traditional approach to the organization of care called *task allocation*. Task allocation simply meant that the nurse's work focused on tasks rather than patients. For instance one nurse would be responsible for all of the wound dressings on the ward; one would be responsible for the ward rounds; whilst another (usually the most junior) nurse would help in the bathroom. In the primary nursing system, a single nurse – called the primary nurse – is responsible for every aspect of the nursing care of a given patient; she assesses the patient on admission, develops the care plan, and is responsible for the delivery of care and its evaluation. The primary nurse is assisted in this work by one or more associate nurses. Advocates of primary nursing claim that this approach produces care of a higher standard than the task allocation approach.

Before leaving our discussion of this aspect of the nurse's role, it is worth considering one more contribution which nurses often make to the running of the health service – the management of change. To the outsider, the National Health Service may appear to be a relatively stable and dependable part of the nation's life. In fact, its systems and structures have been the subject of enormous change in recent years. Some of these changes have been the result of government directives and recommendations, whilst others have been brought about by the public's changing expectations of the NHS. In addition, nursing research has offered new insights into the processes of care delivery. Each of these issues has produced changes in the way in which nursing care is delivered, and nurses often play an important role in introducing and managing these changes. The management of the process of change is an important part of the role of many adult nurses.

CONCLUSION

If you choose to make your career in adult nursing, you will find that the job is rewarding, demanding, intellectually challenging, physically tiring, occasionally difficult, sometimes repetitive, and generally satisfying. Remember that adult nursing is the branch of the profession with the greatest number of practitioners. Do not restrict your picture of the job to the traditional hospital environment – there is a huge variety of posts within the field, and there may well be one to satisfy your particular interests and skills.

EXERCISE

The impact of illness
1. Imagine that you wake up one morning to find that you have lost all sensation and power in your right hand (assuming that you are right handed). Think about the impact that this would have on your day. What would you be unable to do that you normally are able to do quite easily? What effect would it have on your ability to do your work? How would you feel about it? Would it change the contribution that you make to your family or household? Make a list of all these things.
2. Now imagine that you are a nurse responsible for the care of such a person. Consider and list some of the ways in which you could help them to compensate for their disability, in such a way that they are able to maintain their independence.

CHAPTER 5
Nursing people with learning disabilities/mental handicaps

Peter Birchenall

INTRODUCTION

Learning disability nursing has developed from a unique institutional background which has its origins in the Victorian era of large asylums, many housing in excess of a thousand people with varying types and degrees of disability. Over the years, this group of people has endured labelling and stigma unlike any other section of the population, being described as mentally defective, mentally subnormal, mentally handicapped, and more recently as people with learning disabilities. It took many years, several important inquiries, and a number of influential reports before care in the community became a reality and long-stay mental handicap hospitals were confined to history.

Resulting from the rapid demise of institutional care, the role of nursing, as well as other occupational groups associated with long-stay hospitals, is undergoing dramatic change. The range of skills required of the nurse working in the community is sophisticated and must take into account not only the person with a learning disability, but her family also. In those cases where the person lives at home, members of the family usually provide the day-to-day care, being supported by locally based community learning disability services. These services, which have a health and social service focus, offer round-the-clock expert advice and practical help from a range of highly skilled practitioners such as nurses, specialist doctors, general practitioners, physiotherapists, occupational therapists, psychologists, social workers and dieticians.

Another important area of care provision is the small community unit or house where a homelike environment is provided for groups of people with learning disabilities, supported by nurses and other carers. Nurses work as part of a team, similar to the way that family-based care is delivered. Consequently, caring for people with a learning disability in small group settings is an activity requiring a wide understanding of the work that colleagues from other disciplines actually do.

There are essential differences between the role of a nurse who works as a member of the primary health care team, or community learning disability team, and one who provides care in a small group home; these differences are discussed later. In practical terms, wherever the skills of learning disability nursing are employed they must take into account the entire health care needs of the person, which range across physical, social, intellectual, emotional and spiritual aspects of daily living activities. At this stage it is pertinent to explore the nature of these skills, followed by an example of how they may be applied in practice by considering an actual case study of community living in the person's own home.

THE SKILLS OF LEARNING DISABILITY NURSING

The learning disability nurse is educated and trained to provide a competent service from a number of different perspectives. The nursing process, with its four main headings of assessing the person's needs, followed by planning, implementing and evaluating the care provided, forms a basis for understanding the skills necessary for effective nursing. From the outset, student nurses are taught the skills of communication and basic counselling, which are fundamental to all nursing practice and can be adapted to suit special circumstances. For example, sign language is quite often used with learning disabilities because, in some cases, it is the principal form of communication by the person with a learning disability. Counselling becomes specialist for example, when the nurse is working with a person who has been bereaved. People with profound learning disabilities do not always display grief overtly, and a sensitive, caring nurse, who understands what the person is experiencing, will give expert help and support when and where it is required. The necessity for grief counselling to be an essential part of learning disability nursing is widely accepted.

Physical caring skills remain a central requirement for any nurse, and in the case of learning disabilities these often take on a specialist function. It is not only important for the nurse to know how to care for the physical well being of the person with a learning disability, but also to teach those who provide informal care – mothers, fathers, brothers, sisters and grandparents – how to do the same. Often this entails caring for a person who is epileptic, incontinent, or physically handicapped through immobility or sensory impairment.

The nurse must also be prepared to act in the capacity of advocate for the person with a learning disability, and sometimes the family too; this may entail standing up for the individual's rights in situations where these are being infringed. Knowledge requirements associated with advocacy include: legislation (with special reference to disability), the Citizen's Charter, understanding welfare benefits, having a knowledge of local employment opportunities, and being prepared to educate the general public about learning disabilities as a way of reducing the stigma which still exists in the minds of some people. Successful advocacy often depends upon a teamwork approach to the problem, which is an essential element when providing good quality care. Here again it is important to recognize the role of nursing as part of a team activity.

An increasingly popular area where a nurse can demonstrate skilled care is in the provision of different types of therapy. There are many instances where the learning disability nurse can apply therapeutic skills and knowledge, for example massage and aromatherapy, both of which can be employed in new ways, particularly with people who have behavioural difficulties. Other examples are the relevant skills of physiotherapy and occupational therapy which are usually learned from colleagues within these professions and then applied to nursing practice when required. Music therapy is becoming increasingly important, particularly for group activities. Nurses who work in small group homes are often involved in this type of therapy, usually under the direction of a music therapist; it is fun to do, as well as providing a stimulating form of activity.

Clearly, these skills do not represent an exhaustive list of the nurse's repertoire but serve only to illustrate the specialist nature of this branch of nursing. The following case study describes a little of the life of a man with a profound learning disability. After reading the history, some reflection on his life should provide you with quite a bit of food for thought, both regarding the impact learning disability has and the necessity for the learning disability nurse's skills.

CASE STUDY

John

John, a 25-year-old man, has a profound learning disability which has affected both his intellectual and physical development. He is unable to communicate through normal speech, and cannot move around his environment except when being pushed in a wheel-chair or physically carried by his mother or father. During weekdays he attends a local centre for people with learning disabilities, but when at home John tends to spend much of his time in the lounge on a special piece of equipment called a side-lyer, watching television or listening to music. John's physical comfort, which includes those things we all take for granted such as daily bathing, shaving, using the toilet, dressing and undress-ing, is largely in the hands of his parents. He does go out for weekend trips with his parents in a car specially adapted to suit his purpose.

EXERCISE

From this brief description of John's situation it should be possible for you to reflect on the sort of help and advice that the community learning disability team can offer to his parents and to John himself, in maintaining and improving their collective lifestyle. Take ten minutes to make a list of general things which will cause difficulties for John and his family, and the possible responses of professionals, including the learning disability nurse, to these problems, before continuing to read this section.

From doing this exercise you will have identified what may be described as commonsense things, and indeed much of the work of nursing, including learning disability nursing, is of this common-sense variety. Nevertheless, it requires sensitivity and skill to offer the maximum possible help to clients and their families without being intrusive into their lives. In this context, consider the realities of caring for a person such as John. It is physically and psychologically demanding, particularly on parents and other carers. His parents are likely to be older people, and almost everything they do for John will require continuing physical effort. Breaks from this exertion will be few, and liable to interruption at any time. More than this, there is the demand of coping with ensuring that John does not become frustrated or depressed by the constraints placed on his life. His parents will themselves be no strangers to depression of this kind. Since it is difficult for John to travel, they will hardly ever go away from home together, even to enjoy a meal in a pub. John's lack of mobility makes this difficult enough, but his parents will also be well aware of the attitudes and direct comments of members of the public.

Finally, there will be the constant worry of what will happen to John after they die; most parents of people with learning disabilities live in fear of their children going into institutional care after they die. The learning disabilities nurse will need to work with the whole family and with other carers, to befriend, teach, support, counsel, carry out therapeutic activities, make regular assessments of John's care needs, and ensure the availability of resources to meet these needs. It is indeed a highly skilled and complex job.

WORKING IN SMALL RESIDENTIAL GROUP HOMES

Small group homes for people with learning disabilities offer a caring and supportive environment where health and social care needs can be successfully met. A philosophy of care exists which enables residents to enjoy the normalities of life, far removed from the strict regimentation of institutional living; this is achieved through each person's being valued as a unique human being, treated with dignity and worth. There is no overcrowding, privacy is respected, individuality encouraged, and each person's potential is recognized and developed. Nurses and others who work in this type of environment sleep in the home on a rotational basis. Each carer takes individual responsibility for a resident's general wellbeing, determined by an appropriate, regularly reviewed plan of care, but remains a member of the overall caring team. Group homes are provided by a number of agencies including the health service, social services, voluntary organizations such as MENCAP, and the private sector. Nursing skills are highly valued by these organizations, a fact often reflected when they advertize posts for carers.

By now you will have gathered that gaining expertise in learning disability nursing demands a lot of dedication and application to academic study and practical skills development. You will also have discovered from an earlier part of the book that the route to gaining a nursing qualification in this field follows a similar pattern to other branches of nursing. The next part of the chapter discusses in greater detail the work pattern of the nurse in a changing environment of care.

EXPLORING THE ROLE

The theoretical concept upon which care is planned and delivered is known as 'normalization'. The concept of normalization is somewhat difficult to understand and its complexities are beyond the scope of this chapter. Simply put, it is a process by which people who have lived for many years in institutional care are given access to a normal living environment. Whatever handicap or disability they may have is secondary to their status as people with equal right of access to those services enjoyed by the majority. The application of this process has made nurses and others review their role to meet changing circumstances. The permanence of change is a reality where care in the community is concerned. Nursing has been focused into redefining its role within a culture of community care that calls for the full integration of people with learning disabilities. New patterns of service are being developed, based on the foundation laid by normalization, which entail having equal access to all those things which support an ordinary lifestyle. Responsiveness to need is the principle by which learning disability nurses are governed, and as such it becomes essential for them to be part of a larger network of services, specialist or otherwise. As the memory of institutional care becomes even more distant, it appears likely for community services to be managed locally with ease of access.

HEALTH CARE

The general practitioner will become a focal person in the provision of health care to people with learning disabilities who are living in community-based residential facilities. Many general practitioners are fund holders and this will shape the service offered to their patients, and ultimately will determine the very nature of community care. As part of their advocacy role, nurses have a duty to protect the interests of learning disabled people who live in the community. This can be achieved in part by ensuring that fund holding GPs understand the principles by which health care to this section of the community is delivered. It is on this basis that it becomes important that community learning disability nurses are considered to have equal standing with district nurses and health visitors when determining priorities for competing health care resources.

SOCIAL CARE

Social care represents another growth area of provision and involves the nurse in what is described as interagency work. This means working with social workers, council officials, voluntary organizations, shopkeepers, and possibly local churches and other community resources, in establishing a network of locally based social care. Acceptance of learning disabled people into a community sometimes raises difficulties, and the nurse is well placed to smooth the pathway when faced with objections from local residents. From my own experience, I can relate several instances where nurses have used their communication skills to bring about attitude change in people who opposed the siting of community living accommodation in their neighbourhood. The 'not in my back yard' syndrome will remain with us for a long time yet, but through education and positive communication it can be reduced. In many cases it amounts to fear of the unknown, which can be resolved by including people from the locality in social events such as barbecues or bonfire night celebrations.

SELF CARE

It is reasonable to say that most people reading this book are able to perform the basics of life with minimum fuss: getting dressed, preparing a meal, washing and bathing unaided, communicating with others, are things we take for granted. Imagine for a moment that you can't do these things, or it takes an age to do simple activities like tying a shoe lace, putting on a tie, going to the shop, or eating in the company of others. These basic social skills are an essential component of daily living, and that is why we learn them early in life from parents and teachers. The term 'learning disabilities' would suggest that acquiring knowledge and skills necessary for leading a normal lifestyle in modern society is, for some, quite difficult. Many people with learning disabilities have poor memory and a limited attention span. Consequently, learning social skills requires repetition, and the breaking down of activities into small, easy to learn parts. Nurses become involved in this aspect of a person's life and this accounts for a substantial part of their work. Now carry out the following exercise.

EXERCISE

Imagine you are going to a local video library to hire a film. Write down every part of what you would do during the trip, the hire of the video and the return trip. Try to anticipate unexpected occurrences. Try to include every aspect of the journey, including things you regard as too obvious to need stating. Now consider the following:

- Imagine you had just arrived in the area.
- Imagine you were from a country which used a different currency.
- Imagine your home country had totally different ideas of how to interact with others, both in words and actions.
  Taking this exercise further, what if:
- You did not understand the concept of money.
- You had no sense of time.
- You could not remember for longer than five minutes.
- You could not use language at all.

Having completed this exercise you will have gained valuable insight into the challenges which face people with learning disabilities in trying to live a normal life. For the learning disabilities nurse, the challenge is to help their clients in meeting these difficulties and overcoming them, through supervision, advocacy, teaching and training, as well as through educating the public and acting as a model of how we can interact with people with learning disabilities.

CONCLUSION

The aim of this chapter has been to give you an impression of nursing in the field of learning disabilities. It is different from other branches of nursing, particularly in the way that care is organized and delivered. It is rare for the nurse to witness dramatic changes in a person's condition – rewards are gained in other ways. For example, there may be an improvement in a person's ability to use eating utensils following many weeks of teaching and role modelling by the nurse. To achieve this step forward involves a high level of skill, patience and belief in the work. The feeling of achievement is exhilarating and has to be experienced in order to gain any real understanding of what nursing in this special area is all about.

EXERCISE

Ask yourself the following questions:

1. Could I work in a field of nursing where reward for effort often takes a lengthy time to materialize?
2. Am I tolerant of other people's prejudices against mental and physical handicap?
3. Do I hold the view that people with a learning disability have a right to a normal life with equal access to community services?
4. Would I enjoy working in either a community residential setting, or with a community learning disability team visiting people in their own homes?
5. Do I think that most people with a learning disability can achieve some measure of independence?
   If you answer 'Yes' to these questions it may be worthwhile following up your interest by talking to a practising nurse about the work. You could also make an appointment to talk to a nurse teacher who specializes in this work. Such a person can be found in a college of nursing or a university department of nursing studies.

CHAPTER 6
Nursing people with emotional difficulties/mental illness and promoting mental health

Robert Newell

INTRODUCTION

Perhaps the most misunderstood role in nursing is that of the nurse who works with people experiencing emotional and behavioural difficulties – the Registered Mental Nurse (RMN). To many, mental illness is still taboo, and mentally ill people experience considerable hostility from society, ranging from supposedly humorous comments, to prejudice and disadvantage in jobs, housing and social relationships. Yet time and again it has been demonstrated that, despite the scare stories the press delight in, people with psychological difficulties tend to be quiet, passive and safe to be with. Strangely, it is we, the 'normal' members of society who are responsible for the vast majority of violent behaviour. Perhaps because of this, some radical psychiatrists have suggested that it is we, society, who are insane, whilst those whom we label as mad are in fact the sanest of all.

EXERCISE

Before we continue with this chapter is a good time to examine your own views about people with a mental illness. Consider what we mean by mental illness by attempting to conjure up in your mind a portrait of a mentally ill person. Examine this portrait and ask what it says about your own preconceptions about mental illness and normality.

This labelling of the mentally ill has a certain parallel with some attitudes towards those who nurse them. It is often difficult for families, friends, and even other nurses to understand why we should want to spend so much of our time with 'insane' people. Typically, there are two stereotypes of the mental health nurse. We are, apparently, all kind, caring listeners who can deal understandingly with the depths of human misery and mental suffering or, by contrast, we have evolved the thickest of skins to enable us both to deal with such misery without being affected by it, and to deal with the aggressive, disruptive and destructive behaviour associated with stereotypes of the mentally ill. However, since such stereotypes of the mental health nurse remain current, even within nursing, those who are considering mental health nursing need to be aware of them. If nursing with people with learning disabilities is of low status within nursing, mental health nursing runs it a close second.

A further preconception about mental health nursing is that, whilst it takes a special kind of person to do it (caring, tolerant, hard, controlling, and so on), it does not take any particular skill. This is the view that, since the majority of the mental health nurse's work involves listening and talking, anyone can do it, provided they have the necessary personal attributes. It has even been suggested that these attributes cannot be enhanced by education and training, but are unchanging parts of our personality.

The truth of mental health nursing is both more mundane and more complex than the stereotypes described above. There is no doubt that many people come into mental health nursing because they believe they will be effective in caring for and dealing with people experiencing mental distress. They may even regard this as little more than an extension of the caring role they have carried out with friends and family at times of distress. However, being a mental health nurse goes beyond this. In the past, the regime of care for mentally ill people was primarily custodial, and psychiatric nurses were the main providers of this care. More recently, the notion of offering psychological and social, as well as drug treatments has become the prevailing trend, even amongst psychiatrists. Additionally, a greater emphasis is now placed on prevention and treatment in the community. The preparation of mental health nurses has to enable them to meet these challenges.

In consequence, mental health nursing is now a skilled speciality within the profession, with a system of education geared to prepare students to become part of an integrated team working with people with psychological problems. Education will consist of elements of counselling, a grounding in psychology and sociology, in-depth knowledge of psychological disorders and their various treatments (including drug and other physical treatments), as well as an under-standing of the work of the other professional and voluntary organizations involved with people with psychological difficulties. The emphasis is generally on working *with* the client, rather than *caring for* her, and mental health nurses strive to maintain the inde-pendence of their clients. They require considerable knowledge of ethical issues, and indeed, mental health nurses have consistently been at the forefront of 'conscientious objection at work', because of the sometimes controversial treatments (e.g. electro-convulsive therapy (ECT), behaviour modification) with which they and their clients are involved.

HOSPITAL SETTINGS

Although there has recently been a much-publicized move towards the care of mentally ill people in the community, a good deal of mental health nursing and mental health nurse training still takes place in hospitals. For instance, most of the specialities within mental health care are still hospital-based. Mother and baby units, therapeutic community work, forensic psychiatry, intensive rehabili-tation and much child and adolescent care tend to take place on an in-patient basis. In addition, people suffering from particularly acute psychological problems are most likely to be cared for in hospi-tal, at least in the first instance. This is especially likely if the individuals concerned are thought to be at risk of suicide or of harming others because of their problems. As a matter of fact, a recent study showed that people with extremely acute mental health problems can be managed as effectively in the community as in hospital. This way of managing their difficulties is also likely to lead to less disruption of their lives. However, in mental health, as in other aspects of health care, ways of organizing treatment are slow to change, and it is likely that routine care of the acutely mentally ill in the community will not become the norm for some years to come.

As a result, mental health nurses, whether in training during their branch programmes or as newly qualified staff nurses can still often expect to spend considerable time working in hospital settings, either on wards or special units such as day hospitals, where clients come each day for medication, counselling, occupational therapy and other treatments. On the wards, the routine is little different from that of the general wards, with the landmarks of mealtimes, administration of medications, the familiar organization of morning, afternoon and night shifts and the ward reports, during which nurses from one shift hand over the care of clients to those of the next. It is now quite usual, as in general nursing, for one trained nurse to assume overall responsibility for the care of a patient or group of patients, with others, often untrained care assistants or nurses in training, acting as associates in this care, under the system known as primary nursing. The idea here, as in general nursing, is to prevent fragmentation of patient care. In mental health nursing, primary nursing as a method of organizing care may be specially beneficial, if it helps clients to build rapport with a particular primary nurse. However there have so far been very few studies which show that primary nursing, however popular with nurses, confers any greater benefit to patients than older, more traditional ways of managing care.

The major difference from general nursing, for the ward-based mental health nurse, is the absence of any set routine to the day, since there are, in most cases, no physical tasks of care to be performed. In the case of the acutely distressed person, or the older mentally ill person, it may well be that the nurse will be involved in helping with physical care, but this is the exception rather than the rule in mental health work. Most of the time is spent sitting with clients, talking, observing, engaging in activities, and much of this work is extremely unstructured, responding spontaneously to opportunities to build relationships with clients. The following extract from a senior student's 'reflective diary' of ward experience describes a typical day on an acute admission ward.

CASE STUDY

Jan's diary for 21st January 1994 *(the names have been changed)*
8.00 a.m. Finished report. I am going to look after Harry and Jane today. Spend 10 minutes planning what to do.
8.15 a.m. Go round bedrooms, making sure clients know it is

time to get up. Wake up Roy, an older man, who would stay in bed till dinner if you let him. Roy has been here for 15 years now and is due to be transferred to the community. He doesn't want to go, and plays up when anyone suggests it to him.

8.20 a.m. Sit in day room with four or five patients. Feel at a bit of a loose end.

9.00 a.m. Patients go to breakfast. Usually I go into the daily planning meeting, but today I go down with Jane, who has anorexia, to support her as she tries to eat something (and also to encourage her, make a note of what she eats and make sure she doesn't sneak off to vomit afterwards). Jane knows this, but we get on OK about it.

10.00 a.m. Slow breakfast with Jane, as it usually is. We agree to meet up at 11.00 for a counselling session. I will talk to Jane mainly about her feelings about the weight she has put on recently. Jane now weighs in at 6st 4lbs.

10.30 a.m. Meet with Harry to agree a time to take him out. Harry is very frightened to go out by himself, following a mugging last year, and has also been severely depressed since then, the reason he has come into hospital.

11.45 a.m. Very tiring session with Jane. I do find it difficult listening to her talking about her body. She obviously hates the way she looks so much, now that she is putting on weight again, and it is very hard to know what to say. I will discuss the session with Jo (her primary nurse), who has made a speciality of eating disorders, and we will meet with Jane at the end of the week to revise her plan of care.

1.30 p.m. Go to the local shops with Harry. He is very nervous, and it is quite tiring to be with him and work with his anxieties. I remind him continually that the feelings of fear will pass, provided he stays out long enough, and ask him to give me examples from his life of where he has been afraid and got over it. He is able to do this and calms a bit, but is obviously still very afraid. Still, he manages to stay out for the agreed length of time and reports that his anxiety has gone down from 8/10 to 6/10 during the afternoon.

3.00 p.m. Write up notes in patient records. Sit in day room chatting to patients till end of shift.

As you can see, there are considerable gaps during the day, when Jan would chat or help the clients to keep occupied. This is not the case on all wards, and some are run in a highly structured way. For instance, Roy might, in other circumstances, have been cared for in a specialized rehabilitation ward to prepare him for re-entry into the community. Here he would have experienced tuition and training in tasks concerned with daily living and social skills, so that he could look after himself more effectively on leaving hospital. The plan of care for Roy would be jointly negotiated between Roy himself, his primary nurse and her associates, and other members of the ward team (occupational therapist, doctor, psychologist), with the result that a 'programme' of activities designed to promote his independence would be arranged covering each day. Similarly, Harry's walks could have formed part of a highly structured behaviour therapy programme taking up much of his waking time, all geared towards helping him overcome his anxieties and supervised by a nurse skilled in behavioural techniques. Nevertheless, a great deal of mental health work with in-patients is not characterized by this level of structure, and it often takes time to adapt to working in the informal way described here. There is a trend towards more structured, goal-centred care for people with mental health problems, but, as in the example of community care for the acutely disturbed, old ways of managing mental health change slowly, and much informal, unstructured caring still goes on. Ward nurses can still expect to spend time simply sitting with clients and finding their own way of working without formal structures.

MENTAL HEALTH NURSING IN THE COMMUNITY

Harry was admitted to the ward because of severe depression, rather than to help with his anxiety about going out. Nowadays, it would be very unusual to be admitted to hospital for treatment of agoraphobia, but in-patient treatment used to be quite a normal approach to this and many other such difficulties. It was noted earlier that mental health care is now centred on the community, and it is here, in community mental health centres, outpatients' clinics and the client's own home that the bulk of care is carried out.

The move towards community care is one which has had an impact on all areas of nursing, but the principal change has undoubtedly been in mental health nursing where, since the mid-1950s, there has been continuing closure of the large old mental hospitals. These closures began with the rundown of so-called 'long-stay' beds, where clients or patients might have been looked after for 20 years or more, long after the acute phase of their illnesses had passed. However, during the 1950s, a whole range of new and powerful psychoactive drugs was developed, with the result that treatment became briefer and more effective. As a result, long-term admissions to the old psychiatric hospitals were no longer required, with the further consequence that the risk of institutionalization was greatly reduced. The large mental hospitals gradually came to be used only for the most difficult cases and for the continuing care of those who had lived in the hospital for most of their lives.

At the same time, thinking about psychiatry was changing, and the notion of asylum from the world during times of psychological distress fell into disuse, to be replaced by the belief that it was better to face such difficulties in the situations where they occurred, a belief which is still current in today's psychological care. More than this shift in belief, the matter of convenience arose. The large hospitals were often set in large grounds in the country, miles from the homes of those who became patients. This led to difficulty for relatives visiting the hospital, and for patients having leave to visit their homes. Even a trip to the shops could become a major excursion from some of the more isolated hospitals. Finally, the large mental hospitals were extremely uneconomical to run, often being little less than small towns in their own right, with all the support facilities this entailed. Money which might have been better spent on patient care went into upkeep of the property.

Today, many acute services for people with mental health problems are housed in special wards in large district general hospitals, which are managed little differently from, say, a cardiac or renal ward. All these psychiatric wards will maintain close links with the surrounding community, often through the work of community psychiatric nurses (CPNs). As with hospital closure, the work of these nurses began in the 1950s, but has considerably expanded since then. Originally envisaged as nurses who would keep a continuing watching brief on patients discharged form the long-stay wards, CPNs (now often called community mental health nurses) quickly expanded their role to include the care of more acutely distressed people. During the 1970s, the most crucial change in their work came with attachment to general practitioner surgeries, taking a caseload of clients direct from the GP as well as from hospital consultant psychiatrists. In essence, this remains the way in which CPNs work today, although they have also developed a large educational component to the job.

The CPN will typically have a caseload of over twenty people, some of whom will have long-term mental health problems. Apart from support and guidance in returning to society, these individuals will often need help with continuing to take the medication which forms part of their continuing care. The CPN will offer this help and guidance, and will also monitor side-effects of the drugs and help the person to recognize if their symptoms are returning. Generally speaking, however, many of the CPN's clients will never have been inside a mental hospital, and will have been referred as the result of some personal crisis requiring counselling and professional support. Many CPNs go on to take specialist training in one or more forms of counselling or therapy, in order to provide a better service to this large client group. Apart from this face-to-face contact with clients, the CPN is also involved in considerable liaison work, for example with general practitioners, hospital wards, social services and the courts. Chris, a CPN working in an urban area, summed up his role like this.

CASE STUDY

Conversation with Chris

Well it is a varied job, I'd have to say. Take today, for instance, I went into a school to do a teaching session with some teenagers about stress. I had been asked to do this by staff in the school, whom I'd run a stress management workshop for a few months earlier. They felt their pupils would get something out of it, too, particularly those coming up to exams, so they found a slot in the timetable for me the next term. It's something I enjoy doing, that kind of preventive work, although it would be good to have had some training in teaching.

Anyway, because I was doing this at 10 o'clock, I came into the office first and caught up a bit on the paperwork. Normally, I might come into the office about half eight and then go straight out again on a visit, or, if it's on my way, visit a client on the way in to work. I try and get in at some point each day, though, to collect messages and so on. After the class at the school, I drove off to (name of town) to see an older gentleman. He's a great bloke. Been in and out of hospital for many years. They say he has schizophrenia, but he doesn't often get any symptoms now. I'm helping him at the moment because he's quite depressed and finds talking helps. I'll probably see him two or three times more.

Then I had a clinic visit at the local health centre. I saw three clients there this afternoon. The first was a woman who was bereaved three years ago but hasn't been able to adjust to it. Then I saw a young bulimic girl, and finally a man who is quite severely depressed. I use a broadly cognitive therapy (a highly focal form of counselling) approach with these clients, and they seem to be responding, although it's often difficult to know if you are doing any good.

Then, that was about it for the day. There are times when you would like to do more, of course, and get frustrated because of the wasted time spent travelling, but the thing about this job is that you have a lot of freedom to organize your work and to make your own decisions, and you do feel as if you're making a difference to the people you come into contact with. I hope to go on with the cognitive therapy – do a training course, and so on. Then, hopefully, I'll be able to approach the job with more expertise.

Although many CPNs work in the community after just the basic training as RMN, the more senior practitioners, like Chris, have often undertaken a further qualification (a certificate, or more recently diploma, course for CPNs) to enhance their understanding of working in the community. It is by no means unusual to find mental health nurses who have undergone considerable further training in order to help them enrich their understanding of their particular area of specialization.

SPECIALIST PRACTICE IN MENTAL HEALTH

In mental health nursing, the major areas of specialization include behaviour therapy, working with children and adolescents, working with drug- and alcohol-dependent people, working in secure settings, for which specialist courses are available, organized and validated by the ENB. These courses aim to prepare RMNs to work within the specialized areas with a greater degree of knowledge and skill, but are not a requirement to work in the areas. All the courses require participants to gain core skills in areas such as nursing research as well as in the specialized skills they will need for the particular client group involved. An amount of extension to the nursing role is involved in every case, with behaviour therapists having the greatest degree of autonomy and flexibility, and working as independent practitioners. Advancing in a particular speciality of mental health nursing generally requires the possession of some further relevant qualification.

Apart from these ENB organized qualifications, mental health nurses have undertaken a very broad range of formal qualifications related to their areas of special interest but without any agreed status within the profession. These qualifications can help both in gaining skills and in securing promotion. A key example is counselling, where dozens of organizations offer qualifications at a variety of levels, from basic introductions to Master of Arts level. Many of these courses are completely unregulated, with the consequence that it is difficult for the intending participant to get an idea both of what skills are likely to be gained and how acceptable the qualification is likely to be within mental health nursing.

More difficult still, there are many people, both inside and outside nursing, practising counselling and therapy on the basis of having completed courses which are intended to offer only awareness of the area, not a certificate to practise. The same is true of many of the alternative and complementary therapies, which are also finding popularity within mental health nursing. Although many major organizations offering counselling and counselling training now offer registration with their organizations and, through affiliation, with the United Kingdom Council for Psychotherapy (UKCP), the problem does not stop there, since any organization can offer registration, and, in order to affiliate to UKCP there is little requirement that any *effectiveness* of the therapy be demonstrated. As a result, nurses seeking further training of this kind need to be extremely circumspect in interpreting the claims of the various therapies, and in suggesting such therapies to clients. Courses validated by major institutions, such as universities, are most likely to be accepted within the profession, although, once again, this does not necessarily imply any therapeutic effectiveness. However, the strongest courses will include some critique of their methods.

CONCLUSION

Mental health nurses have taken the role of psychological caring to the farthest point of any of the branches of nursing. Although many elements of physical caring still remain, particularly when working with the older client, this is usually secondary to the provision of psychological care. This makes mental health nursing particularly challenging since, if it is done well, it requires us to examine constantly our own perceptions about such notions as loss, bereavement, anxiety, fear, responsibility – even ideas about right and wrong and the nature of 'normal' and 'abnormal' behaviour, thoughts and feelings. Mental health nurses are often involved in working with people who do not even share our most basic beliefs about the way the world works. The great quest in mental health nursing is for the ability to be open to these different experiences and to remain sufficiently resilient to cope with them, whilst at the same time handling the considerable practical difficulties involved in addressing these issues in a rapidly changing society which would often rather forget about people with mental health problems.

EXERCISE

1. Having read this chapter, return to the exercise we carried out right at the beginning. Briefly carry it out again – consider what we mean by mental illness by attempting to conjure up in your mind a portrait of a mentally ill person and examine the portrait and ask what it says about your own preconceptions about mental illness and normality – has your portrait changed? If so, how? What do the changes say about you?

2. Every couple of weeks, a case arises of a person who comes to the attention of the media owing to mental illness, either through committing a crime or because of some unusual behaviour. Go to the library and look at back issues of popular newspapers for examples of this. Get out the film *Psycho* from your video library. Make some notes about the way in which the media tackle mental health issues.

3. We all come into contact with distressed people during our daily lives. Perhaps you have a friend, neighbour or relative who has had a time of distress, for instance through an exam disappointment, a break-up in a relationship, or even a bereavement. Consider the effect *their* distress had on *you*.

4. What do you do to cope with the emotions of others?

Further reading

Brooking, J., Ritter, S. A. H., and Thomas, B. L. (1992) *A Textbook of Psychiatric and Mental Health Nursing*. Edinburgh: Churchill Livingstone.

Goffman, E. (1968) *Asylums*. Harmondsworth: Penguin.

Laing, R. D., and Estherson, A. (1964) *Sanity, Madness and the Family*. Harmondsworth: Penguin.

Marks, I. M. (1980) *Living With Fear*. New York: McGraw-Hill.

CHAPTER 7
Nursing with children and their families in sickness and health

Lesley Sheldon

INTRODUCTION

What is different about nursing children? Are they simply small adults with similar needs? Is the care required similar to that of adult clients, or the elderly? Are children with health problems that require surgical treatment the same as adults and thus require similar treatment and care? In earlier times, childhood was indeed thought of as an incomplete and inadequate form of the adult state. If this is the case why is there such a need for specialist practitioners who are skilled and dextrous in this unique field of practice?

Children's nursing is a speciality that is extremely complex and challenging. Children vary in age and thus have differing physical and developmental characteristics, but age alone does not dictate the domains of physical, psychological and social development of each individual child. The child's need for intervention by the health professional is continuous from one day old through mid- to late adolescence and the type of intervention required will depend upon the particular needs of the child and her family in health and illness at any given point in time.

To be skilled and competent to nurse children, your training will have given you the knowledge and experience to care for the child as a whole, encompassing his complete physical and emotional wellbeing and not simply the health problem you are preventing, detecting or treating. You will also learn to be extremely skilled in caring for the family, including grandparents, siblings and estranged partners.

You need skills to practise family-centred care, to be in a position to teach families and empower them with your knowledge and skills so that they can take over the care required; and above all you need to be able to recognize that children have rights to be treated as individuals and not as small adults. Children need to be valued for what they are as well as for what they can become. These are the skills which training in children's nursing attempts to provide for you.

THE COMMUNITY

Your work may involve working in the home and community, for example in schools, health centres, creches, youth clubs, where the majority of your interventions will be aimed at preventing or detecting health problems. You might work alongside health visitors undertaking developmental assessments, providing advice regarding child safety and prevention of accidents and also providing immunization. You may decide that you wish to work with older children, perhaps in conjunction with a school nurse continuing with development assessments and accident prevention, but also broader issues such as sexual health and health awareness of the older child and adolescent. However, you may feel that you wish to support families and children at home where the child has either an acute health problem or is recovering from an acute illness. You may act as a resource to the child and family or be involved in giving active care just as you would in hospital, but in the child's home.

Another aspect of home and community nursing is that of caring for the child with special and/or long-term health needs. You may find yourself working in 'special schools' for those children who either have learning difficulties or who have a handicap, or indeed you may be supporting children who have long-term health problems such as asthma, cystic fibrosis, diabetes or eczema in a normal mainstream school. Crucial to your support and care will be identifying family resources and providing families with education and skills to nurture their children from dependence to independence.

As a practitioner working with children in any setting you will learn to be vigilant and attentive, in order to identify those children at risk or potential risk from physical, emotional or social abuse or neglect. You may even decide you wish to specialize in practice in the field of child protection. One thing you will learn is that, although families and carers are essential to the welfare of children, and generally they are best looked after by their families, the welfare of the child is absolutely paramount and their needs are uppermost if there is a conflict between those and carer/parental needs.

The types of children's nurse practitioner described above are based mainly in the home and community settings, although some of their work may take them into hospital or 'acute' settings when an individual child requires such services because the particular stage in her life necessitates hospital care.

HOSPITAL NURSING

You may decide to reverse the balance of acute and community care and spend the majority of your time in hospital, with only a proportion spent at home or in the community. If this is the route you take initially, then again working with children and their families offers an endless variety of opportunities. For example, you may wish to practise as a Registered Children's Nurse in a general ward where children are admitted with acute health problems. Some children may be there as a result of an accident, others may be having emergency surgery. There are those whose admission is a result of a long-term health problem that requires medical treatment and nursing care, and those where admission is chiefly to bring relief and a timely break for parents and carers; where a child has a handicap, for example.

If this doesn't appeal, then you may wish to work in accident and emergency, but be solely responsible for planning the care of children brought in as casualties, to meet their needs and those of their families. This may be very traumatic, as you will be involved in supporting families through grief and shock following an accident or death of their beloved child, but you will need to have proficient first aid and emergency skills to cope both with simple cuts, bruises, grazes and with children who need urgent emergency care involving the use of specialized equipment. Part of the challenge of nursing in general, and children's nursing in particular, is to be able to integrate these personal and practical skills. As a result, these skills are heavily emphasized during training.

An alternative to accident and emergency nursing which also utilizes these skills is theatre and anaesthetic nursing. Again it takes special skills and knowledge to enable a child safely to progress through anaesthesia to recovery, attending to both psychological and physical needs (for example, keeping the child's and family's emotions intact and ensuring that wounds are free from infection!).

Children's intensive care is a speciality that demands humour and rigorous attention to detail. The cause of the child's visit will result in great physical stress to the child and emotional stress to the family/carers. Each child and family has unique needs and resources, and the children's intensive care nurse needs to combine technical interventions and child- and family-centred approaches, to enable the child either to recover to his maximum potential or to die a peaceful death.

Children's nurses also specialize in 'Special Care Baby Units'. If this is a field which interests you, you will be involved not only in providing care of a highly specialized nature to very sick newborn and premature infants, but also in supporting a nervous mum or dad in getting used to their new family member, within the context of extreme worry and uncertainty about the child's future. There are also specialist areas where your skills of children's nursing will be highly valuable combined with specialist skills such as nursing children with cancer, AIDS, heart problems and many difficulties requiring a combination of high level technical skills and a sympathetic approach to family relationships and emotions. Your initial training in children's nursing will lay a foundation upon which to build these specialist skills.

QUALITIES OF CHILDREN'S NURSES

What are the rewards of nursing children and working with them? As suggested in chapter 1, when pressed, many would-be student nurses would say that wanting to be a nurse has something to do with wanting to help people or look after them. Likewise, many potential students of children's nursing would state that they 'liked children' or 'were good with them'. These are fundamental to the creation of a good children's nurse. To work with children you must enjoy being with them, love having them around and, more importantly, understand and respect them. Nurses training to work with children are expected to undertake a holistic study of childhood – physical, intellectual, emotional, social, cultural and spiritual. They also study attitudes towards childhood in other times and cultures, and the religious beliefs and practices and political ideologies which inform and influence current attitudes. Students of children's nursing are also expected to read books written for children, watch television and video, read comics and spend time at Brownie and Scout clubs, playgrounds, youth groups and schools, watching, listening and learning. After all, how can one be expected to identify, assess and care for a sick 5-year-old when the behaviours and experiences of the well 5-year-old are unknown.

Since in Britain only 28 per cent of the population are children, likewise only a small minority of nurses are children's nurses. This has implications for the student of children's nursing. She has to be politically aware, assertive, have a thorough knowledge of her subject, health economics and health influences generally at local, national and international level. She needs to be prepared to lead solid discussion and debate concerning child health and children's nursing. Above all she will need the knowledge and skills to act as advocate for the vulnerable clients whom she is charged with serving.

THE EXPERIENCE OF CHILDREN'S NURSING

Children are cared for at home for as long as possible or return home quickly after a stay in hospital. For the child in hospital, it is now recognized that if the child's psychological needs are not being met, then we are at risk of causing emotional harm and, as a result, we encourage mothers or significant others to stay with the child in hospital. If this is not possible then unrestricted visiting is encouraged and children are cared for by their own 'special nurse' – the number of different nurses is kept to a minimum and, in some hospitals, this has extended to the 'primary nursing' concept, where a Registered Children's Nurse has full responsibility for that child from admission through to discharge, 24 hours a day. Obviously, she is not on duty for all that time, but she retains overall responsibility for the plan of care.

Children's psychological needs are also met through play and play therapy. These are crucial elements of the children's nurse's role, working alongside a trained play therapist. Children need to play to occupy and entertain themselves, but also to prepare them for certain treatments and procedures. Play is also valuable to enable nurses to understand children's fears and feelings, as the child may express these during play.

Families need support and care too. Admitting a child to hospital can often cause more distress among the parents than the child, leaving the parents with feelings of anxiety, guilt, fear and self-blame. These feelings, if not addressed by the skilled children's nurse, may transmit to the child, delaying recovery. As one parent said to me: 'I always remember the day Sam was diagnosed with leukaemia, I remember exactly what the nurse did and said, her eyes said so much! Even then I knew Sam would be treated as an individual – not as a leukaemic, a statistic.'

Children's nurses, then, are flexible people who offer care in a variety of settings, constantly liaising and working with parents to care for children. The nurse exercises considerable responsibility and judgement, considering and supporting the family as a whole.

CASE STUDY

Rebecca

A week before her first birthday, Rebecca started to cough during the night. Her parents, a young Australian couple visiting relations in London, quickly called in their GP, who diagnosed suspected meningitis and arranged for the child to be admitted to a local children's ward. Rebecca was normally a very happy, active girl, but by the time of admission was both subdued in manner and physically exhausted. She had a series of blood tests and a lumbar puncture, which confirmed the diagnosis. As a result, Rebecca had to be placed in a room by herself, since she was potentially infectious to others, and given antibiotics through an intravenous drip for ten days. During the early days of her illness, she remained very ill, and also needed feeding through the drip, as well as continuing monitoring of her temperature and other vital signs. Fortunately, she made a full recovery from this potentially fatal disease.

The children's nurses on the ward provided both physical care and skilled observation and treatment for Rebecca. Much more than this, however, they involved her parents at all times. Rebecca's illness had major effects on her family, which the nurses helped them to deal with. Her parents were very upset by Rebecca's having to go into hospital and fearful about the future. After admission, during the lumbar puncture test, which is both frightening and unpleasant, Rebecca had to be held down. Tina, her mother, became very tearful and unhappy, but was able to talk to the nurse about her feelings. After a while, fear gave way to anger, and Tina came to blame herself for not spotting signs of illness earlier. The nurse helped her talk through this.

Involving Tina and her husband in caring for Rebecca helped

them feel they were being useful and helped preserve their relationship with their daughter. As well as this, being part of the care team helped them gain in confidence, and allayed some of their fear about the disease Rebecca was fighting. The nurses even involved Sandra, Rebecca's older sister, trying to help her to understand what was happening as far is she was able to at 3 years old.

For Rebecca, who had to endure her first birthday in hospital, this could all have been a traumatic part of her childhood. The constant presence of her parents and the nurses, who took time to explain what they were doing through play, seemed to help Rebecca, and there were no apparent ill-effects. The main aim of the nurses, apart from physical and medical care, was to preserve the normal aspects of Rebecca's family life and relationships as far as possible. Today Rebecca is 4 years old, with nothing to suggest she was ever acutely ill. She is a happy, loving girl, close to her parents and sister. Her parents still send a card to the ward on Rebecca's birthday and at Christmas.

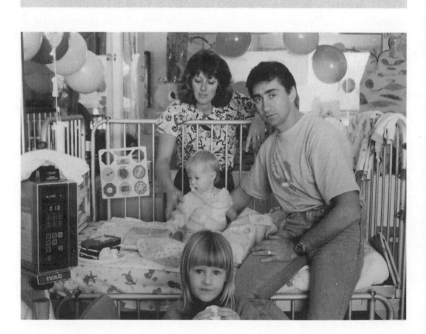

Rebecca, on her 1st birthday, admitted with meningitis

Today's parents expect to have a healthy baby and to provide a safe and happy future for their children. When a child has an illness, no matter how mild or serious, parents find the situation hard to accept and cope with. The whole family is deeply affected; they find themselves in a strange new world. Nurses need to be strong and sensitive to face their own emotions and accept their own feelings and values, so that they can support the family. Nursing children is about facing one's values and beliefs head on – parents, carers and families seek your support, whilst children may challenge it.

EDUCATION OF CHILDREN'S NURSES

The majority of children's nurses are today educationally prepared to diploma level by studying the children's nursing branch of Project 2000. This provides them with the unique opportunity to translate theories of nursing and those related to nursing (e.g. psychology, sociology, biological science, ethics, law research, information technology and nursing theory studies), studied during their common foundation programme (see chapter 2), into the art and science of children's nursing. Once in the branch programme, they are exposed to children in all the settings described earlier, where they progress through a variety of roles from being a reflective observer to becoming a supervized practitioner. At all stages they are expected to reflect, clarify, define, redefine and evaluate nursing as applied to particular client groups (e.g. children in accident and emergency or children undergoing a six-week developmental assessment).

Having achieved the diploma and award as a Registered Nurse (Children's), qualified nurses are expected to continue to update their academic knowledge and practical skills in their field of specialization. For example, BSc courses in children's nursing/child health are becoming popular, as are masters level degrees in nursing children.

There are some colleges of nursing that prepare nurses for registration by way of a degree route. Typically this is of four years duration, although it is possible that this might be reduced to three years in some settings in the future. There are other routes of entry, particularly for the adult nurse or the nurse registered to care for clients with mental health problems or learning disabilities wishing to undertake a further nursing registration. Many colleges are providing a fast-track, modified branch programme for such students: the length of time for this will vary but will normally be one calendar year.

PERSONAL COSTS

As suggested earlier, children's nursing is not easy. All the difficulties present in other branches of nursing occur in children's nursing, yet there are additional challenges and responsibilities created by the varied developmental stages and social status of the child. How does a six-month-old infant tell you he is in pain? How do you explain to a 3-year-old that he needs a circumcision, and that this will necessitate coming to a strange environment and to be cared for by strange people? How does a 5-year-old associate a broken leg with pain and being in hospital? How do you explain to a 4-year-old that his tummy pain is not caused by him being naughty? How do you prepare a 14-year-old with leukaemia to go back to school? How do you support a grieving family when their eldest son has been killed in a cycling accident? How do you reassure a family that their daughter's meningitis was not their fault and give them the skills to care for her in hospital?

Nursing children is hard, both cognitively and emotionally. To nurse a child and family through what may potentially be an extremely vulnerable and stressful time – to be allowed to enter the private world of that child and his significant family members is a stressful privilege, but a privilege, nonetheless. To be able to share in the privilege, but withstand the stress, children's nurses need to have good – and I mean really good – support networks: hobbies, family and friends; and to know where work ends and home life begins. Children's nursing is hard, but it is a lot of fun too!

EXERCISE

1. Make a list of 10 differences between nursing children and nursing adults. Don't forget to include children's families and their needs, as well as the needs of the children themselves.
2. What implications do these differences have in terms of skills? Examine what you will need to do differently when nursing children from when nursing adults.

SECTION 4
PROGRESSING AS A NURSE

This section is intended not only for the person considering nursing for the first time, but also for the trained nurse who is wondering where to go next. The intending student will find much information here about future directions in nursing, and we hope this will enrich your understanding of the many facets of the nursing life and give you some broad notions of how your career might go in future years if you decide to undertake nurse training. For the trained nurse who has perhaps gone through the process of consolidation of practice described in the previous section, there may well still be considerable doubt about where her career in nursing is leading.

We have stressed throughout this book that nursing is now a very broadly-based profession, and nowhere is this more apparent than in the role of the specialist clinician. These nurses have developed, through experience and education, an advanced clinical role which allows them a great deal of independence in practice. All nurses are accountable for their practice, but in the case of the nurse specialist, this practice is likely to be extremely far-reaching, and therefore the degree of autonomy and accountability will be that much greater. Specialist nurses now exist across all branches of nursing and continue to push forward the frontiers of nursing clinical knowledge and practice.

Health care in general, and nursing in particular, has moved away from an emphasis on hospital care towards care in the community. The area in which this move has received the greatest publicity is that of mental health and learning disabilities care, where some of the publicity has been unjustifiably negative. At the same time, however, the other disciplines of nursing have strengthened and enhanced a community role which has been part of the fabric of nursing for decades. The change in policy towards community care has led to an increase in the breadth of practice for these experts in community care (e.g. community nurses, health visitors, school nurses, practice nurses) and to increased responsibility. They have responded to these challenges through continuing education and have begun to examine their own practice through structured research into their roles and effectiveness.

Management in nursing was, until recently, a speciality undervalued by many nurses, and by managers from other disciplines. For most nurses, the major division between 'nursing' and 'management' occurs when they leave the clinical setting; at least, it is the perception of students and junior staff that this is the point at which nurses become managers. Yet management is a function of the nurse throughout her career. Even as students we are required to self-manage as we juggle the competing needs of the clinician and the student throughout our pre-registration training. As staff nurses, ward management becomes a significant part of our role, which is increased with further promotion, even if we remain within the clinical arena.

Traditionally nurses had principally managed the work of other nurses, but the NHS is now organized according to a general management structure, where individuals from any professional background (including a large number of managers with no clinical background at all) can manage diverse staff groups. In consequence, many nurse managers argue that it is essential that the nursing profession is adequately represented within the general management structure, so that nursing continues to have a voice in the management of its work, right to the highest level.

As you will know from reading the earlier chapters of this book, nurse education has undergone huge changes. For the nurse teacher, this has led to great dislocations, but also to great challenges. Those of you who are already in training as nurses, or have now qualified, will be familiar with some of the work of the nurse teacher. There are, however, many aspects of the teaching role which are not seen by the student, for example course planning, and the organization of clinical placements and new courses. In a well-run educational establishment most of these elements are hidden from the student and tend only to be noticed when things go wrong! Peter Birchenall is an extremely experienced teacher, and also knows the world of nurse education from the other side, having been an inspector of colleges of nursing for some years. As well as dealing with practical issues surrounding training to be a nurse teacher, he demonstrates how, as with management, the role of the nurse is concerned with teaching from the beginning, and how this role is naturally extended into the formal teaching role of the nurse lecturer.

Research in nursing is a young speciality. Traditionally, the work of nurses had been based either on the theoretical knowledge of other disciplines, or upon custom and practice, often now referred to as 'nursing rituals'. In the United States, nursing research has a comparatively long history. In the UK, we are now defining a research tradition in nursing to carry our practice forward into the next century. We have gone down a route of formal training in research for the profession, so that all nurse training contains at least some element of education in research methods and awareness. Moreover, all theoretical teaching in nursing aims to draw on relevant research. At the moment, opportunities for careers in research are still few, but are increasing all the time. Certainly, nurse researchers are committed to investigating our practice, and are accepted as equal members of research teams. Perhaps more importantly, there is a sense that this is now *our* research; nursing is no longer researched by non-nurses using nursing as their subject matter, and our reliance on research from other disciplines diminishes as our own research abilities increase. Nursing research is now owned by nurses and their clients.

As you will see, there is considerable choice for the experienced nurse. A good many people will not want to go beyond staff nurse level, which itself involves a great deal of skill and sensitivity. For those who do wish to continue their professional development, appropriate decision making at an early stage will certainly speed this process. So, if you are still at the point of starting to think about nursing, please read this section anyway. We intend that reading this section will provide you with a concise guide to these choices. It will also give you some more experience of what nurses do as their careers develop. No doubt, if you are reading this as a trained nurse, you will have had considerable contact with people working in many of the roles which we describe, but this section is definitely for you too, since we offer its chapters as a process for you to go through to inform your decision making about future careers. Since further training and education will almost certainly be a requirement for progressing as a nurse, some of the key aspects of such training are also outlined by the authors.

CHAPTER 8
The nurse as a specialist clinician

Linda Veitch

INTRODUCTION

A number of qualified nurses now choose to specialize in a particular area of nursing and recognize that their basic programme was only the start of attaining knowledge sufficient to become a competent practitioner. There are numerous specialities within nursing and in my previous post, in a continuing education department in a college of nursing, we co-ordinated 38 post-basic courses. With the increasing maze of specialities within nursing it is crucial that you formulate your own career plan.

Over the next few paragraphs, I shall use my own background as an example of one way of going about negotiating the process of career and professional development decision making. I used the 'nursing process' as a framework to aid my decision making with regard to my initial career aspirations. The nursing process is a structured way of making decisions about patient care, but is also readily adaptable to almost any decision-making process. It involves dividing decision making into a cycle of *assessment* of what needs to be done, *planning* of how you will go about doing it, *implementation* of these plans and *evaluation* of what you have done during these three phases. By the time you have amassed some basic post-registration experience as a nurse, you should be familiar with the nursing process as a problem-solving cycle.

Assessment

What aspect of nursing did I most enjoy and why? What were my strengths and weaknesses both personal and professional?

Planning

Aim for a staff nurse position within an intensive care unit (ITU).

Intervention

Compile and submit my curriculum vitae. Prepare for the interview for first staff nurse position ITU.

Evaluation

Successful application: but I quickly recognized that my basic training was inadequate for the position I now held. Therefore, plan to investigate post-basic courses and requirements.

I have not included all the questions that needed to be addressed in my individual case, but try the exercise yourself and see how it works for you. Within my own speciality of intensive care nursing I was fortunate to have numerous career choices in all four major aspects of nursing: management, education, practice and research. To enable me to access this further focus within my speciality, it was necessary to undertake further courses. Therefore, I suggest that you plan your career path and monitor your own job satisfaction. Remember it is never too early or too late to plan your career.

Over the last decade the number of specialities has continued to grow. It is not the aim of this chapter to cover the specialist–generalist debate, but to provide an insight into a few specialities that reflect the breadth of career choices available. As the chapter develops, we will look at scenarios which will highlight the reality of nursing within the specialist environment. Since it is impossible to cover the work of all the specialized fields of nursing within a single chapter, a small range of specialities has been chosen to reflect the range across the four branches of nursing.

At the end of Project 2000 training you will have a diploma in addition to one of the following nursing qualifications:

Adult Nursing, Part 12, UKCC Professional Register.

Mental Health Nursing, Part 13, UKCC Professional Register.

Mental Handicap Nursing, Part 14, UKCC Professional Register, Children's Nursing, Part 15, UKCC Professional Register,

ADULT NURSING

Most nurses opt to train initially in adult nursing, gaining a wide range of experience which, as we saw in chapter 4, then opens up many opportunities for diversification within nursing. In the context of hospital nursing, the impetus for specialization arises from the need to meet the increasing demands made as a result of advances in technology and public expectation. According to the UKCC, specialist practice should indicate that nurses working at this level have the ability to exercise a high degree of clinical decision making and promote research-based nursing care. Of the many avenues available to the adult nurse wishing to specialize, intensive care nursing was one of the first to develop a post-registration course.

CASE STUDY

Career Development – Jan Morris
Jan Morris is a 'D' grade staff nurse on an acute surgical ward. She has been a Registered Nurse for one year. Her qualifications are RN and DipHE. Jan is a valued member of the multidisciplinary team and she has been able successfully to consolidate and develop the knowledge and skills gained during her basic programme.

Today, Jan has an appraisal interview with her ward manager who has actively encouraged Jan's professional development. The purpose of this meeting is to discuss Jan's strengths and weaknesses in her role as 'D' grade staff nurse and also to plan her future career objectives.

Jan has reflected on her clinical experience and has come to the conclusion that she feels frustrated when the patient she has helped to care for becomes more seriously ill and is transferred to the intensive care unit. Jan has questions requiring answers: 'What does an ITU offer that a ward can't?'; 'Why does the patient's family appear to become so impatient with the ward staff when the patient returns?'; 'Rumour has it that ITU nursing is much more stressful than other aspects. True or false?'

The nurse manager has listened to Jan and offers a couple of practical options for her to think about:

a)   Investigate the literature on the positive and negative aspects of intensive care nursing.

b)   Examine the possibility of working some shifts in the ITU with an experienced member of the nursing team.

The nurse manager feels that these options would enable Jan to understand better the role of intensive care nursing within acute nursing.

Within three months Jan has completed six shifts within ITU and finds that she enjoys the 1:1 nurse/patient ratio and the complexity of care, but finds having the family present for most of her shift stressful.

The opportunity to taste ITU enabled Jan to decide that she would request to transfer to the unit as a 'D' grade staff nurse with the long-term aim of undertaking a post-basic course in intensive care nursing. These courses are available throughout the United Kingdom but competition is stiff and the majority of successful candidates will have been working as staff nurses within the speciality for at least six to twelve months, a common pattern within many of the specialities; a period of work is usually required before successful admission to further training. Key exceptions to this rule are those specialities where a further qualification is formally or informally regarded as a licence to practise.

From Jan's perspective, a post-basic course within the critical care field (as well as proven managerial/leadership skills) will almost certainly be regarded as a prerequisite for promotion within the speciality.

MENTAL HEALTH NURSING

There is a wide range of careers/specialities within this branch of nursing. These include behavioural psychotherapy, forensic care, care of the drug- and alcohol-dependent client. In this section we will focus on adult behavioural psychotherapy, using it as an example of how one specialist role in mental health nursing affects the role of the nurse. As you would expect there are appropriate post-basic courses available, of varying duration. The best known is course ENB 650, which enables suitably qualified nurses to become competent in the treatment of patients by behavioural psychotherapy. Nurses trained on the course act as independent clinical practitioners without direction from other professions, and carry out all stages of treatment, assessing, planning, implementing and evaluating the treatment plan formulated in partnership with the client.

There are some specific categories of client disorders treated more than others by the behavioural psychotherapist: phobic disorders, obsessive–compulsive disorders, sexual and habit disorders. Apart from these types of difficulty, 'nurse behaviour therapists', as people trained in this way are called, have expanded their clinical practice to include many other emotional problems and even some physical difficulties for which behavioural treatments have been found to be useful.

Therapy sessions can, however, make considerable emotional demands upon the nurse behaviour therapist. As a therapist you need to develop a trusting relationship with your clients, encouraging them to explore their feelings and behaviour. Clients may require support at any stage of their therapy programme irrespective of where the actual sessions take place.

CASE STUDY

Career Development – Alan Bailey

Alan is a 26-year-old nurse working in an acute admission ward for people with mental health problems. He has become increasingly disillusioned with care in this ward, mainly because he can find little evidence that what he and the other nurses do makes much difference to their patients. He has continued his reading since qualification, and has read a number of papers which indicate the successes of behaviour therapy and cognitive therapy, and also the independent role of the nurse in delivering therapy.

Alan decides to make contact with a nurse behaviour therapist working in the local specialist facility for psychotherapy. This is some miles away, in the nearest major city, since behavioural psychotherapy is a scarce resource.

The behaviour therapist gives Alan a thumbnail sketch of her work, going through an average day:

> I won't say that any two days are ever the same, but here is a rundown of the things I was involved in yesterday. I act as a

consultant about behavioural matters to one of the wards in the local hospital, so I put on occasional study sessions for them. Yesterday, I ran a one-hour session introducing relaxation techniques, which we then followed up with some clinical supervision of individuals they're working with. That took me through till eleven, when I interviewed a new client, with a view to deciding if behaviour therapy would help. In the end, I decided not to take him on, but offered him some brief advice. After lunch, I saw two more clients, a man with agoraphobia, and a woman with a sexual problem; our work involved some talking about the problems, but mainly practical instruction from me and the negotiation of tasks they will carry out between now and our next meetings. Finally, I met with a colleague to discuss a research project we're doing. In behaviour therapy, we spend a good deal of time trying to see if the techniques we use are really useful. Myself and my colleague are developing a new way of dealing with people who self-injure. This is in response to an increase in our referrals of this kind of difficulty. We believe we've made some interesting changes to the way folk with self-injury behaviour are dealt with, and are designing a project which will enable us to examine our interventions with greater precision. The eventual project will take about two years to complete.

She then describes what Alan needs to do if he wants to train as a nurse behaviour therapist. This is difficult, since there are only four ENB 650 courses running in the country. There are, however, many short courses, and she suggests that Alan may undertake one of these, both to get an idea of what behavioural work is like and to increase his chances of being able to get on to a longer course later. Finally, she offers him limited supervision in working with a few clients on his ward using a behavioural approach.

MENTAL HANDICAP NURSING/LEARNING DISABILITY NURSING

A learning disability is generally a permanent condition and can occur in all social groups. The cause can be genetic, environmental or both and may result in sensory or physical impairment. The clients you may care for vary from those with a severe handicap who may be looked after by their parents at home, to those with a mild disability who are capable of living on their own either in a hostel or a shared home. Until recently the main role and function of the qualified nurse has been seen by some as providing a service to clients in hospital. Gradually, this role has been changing and nurses who specialize in learning disability will find themselves working in a variety of settings. Increasingly, it will involve working in the client's own home as a community nurse working with clients/families and social networks.

The aims of the learning disability nurse are to improve and maintain the health and wellbeing of clients and to aid clients to develop skills in order to achieve as much independence and control over their own lives as possible. The nurse will work as part of an integrated health care team including social workers, psychologists and special needs teachers. The change in working patterns for the learning disability nurse has mirrored changes in public attitudes to mental handicap/learning disability. As a result, the profile of learning disability nursing has increased considerably, as has the range of skills required to help people with learning disabilities adapt to a more integrated and independent role in society than would have been thought either appropriate or possible ten or twenty years ago. This increased range of skills has itself given rise to a number of specialist courses within learning disability nursing.

Some of these are aimed at helping nurses themselves adapt to major changes in their working roles, whilst others present new areas of specialization befitting the greater expectations and responsibilities placed on people with a learning disability as they become increasingly accepted as members of the community with a valid part to play. Course ENB 939 deals with 'Moving from the Institution to the Community' and reflects this shift of emphasis specifically, equipping nurses to help their clients deal with the new skills required to move out of long-stay hospital accommodation (where they may have been incarcerated for 50 years or more) into a world which they have only ever known before as occasional visitors.

For even the most able client, this will involve a great deal of adaptation to change. However, the policy of care in the community is common to all and, therefore, the nurse working in this field will need to deal effectively with clients with profound, multiple handicaps. Courses which may help have recently been initiated by the ENB – course N47 ('Mental Illness in Learning Disability') and course N02 ('Challenging Behaviour in Learning Disability'). Indeed, many nurses find that, whilst personally challenging and stressful, both these areas are particularly rewarding, since there is the pleasure of working with people who may, quite literally, be incapable of living in the world, and helping them arrive at a point where, with appropriate support, they can genuinely enjoy a life of their own. More generally, behaviour modification as an approach to the teaching of people with learning disabilities is taught in a range of courses for nurse and other health care workers.

In the following case study a picture is given of someone who lacks quite basic social skills, as a result of institutionalized living.

CASE STUDY

David Pringle
David Pringle is 55 years old and has spent the majority of his life institutionalized in a large Victorian hospital. With the new focus on community care David and his carers are looking at the feasibility of David moving back into the community. There are three key areas that needed to be addressed:

a) David had rarely made a decision for himself – the aim was to encourage David to think for himself at every opportunity.
b) Devise a leisure/work programme – David had previously enjoyed gardening and so it was arranged that David work as a volunteer with a qualified gardener.
c) Enable David to become integrated into his local community – the nurse and David made several outings to the local working men's club where it is hoped that eventually he will be accepted as one of the 'boys'.

David participated with the team in co-ordinating his programme of care. This enabled small skills to be taught in an individual and methodical way.

CHILDREN'S NURSING

As we noted in chapter 6, the prime responsibility of the children's nurse is to support the developing child and her family so that the child's full potential is reached. When children become ill it may not be possible for them to be cared for at home and separation from home can affect their development. Within children's nursing the term family-centred care is used. This simply means that attempts are made to meet the needs of *all* significant family members. In the hospital environment this should mean that the parents are actively encouraged to care for their child.

The post-basic courses available to the children's nurse reflect this family-centred approach to care. Children's nurses have participated in many of the specialist courses designed for adult nurses, and undertaken placements with a particular focus upon the child. In addition, there are post-basic courses available with the children's nurse in mind, including paediatric intensive care, and child and adolescent psychiatric nursing (course ENB 603), on which we will focus in this chapter. This course is suitable for nurses on Parts 3, 4, 5, 6, 8, 13, 14 or 15 of the Professional Register. This requirement ensures that nurses who are planning to undertake the course have previous experience of either nursing children, knowledge of mental health nursing or mental handicap nursing. It is quite unusual in being available to this wide range of nurses, reflecting the breadth of interest within the profession in working with troubled children.

We saw in chapter 6 that work with children is often stressful. Often, this is accentuated within the specialities, and this is particularly true of child and adolescent psychiatric nursing. As an individual contemplating a career move into this field, it is important that you have an interest and affinity with both children and teenagers and an ability to communicate effectively with them during episodes of acute emotional disturbance. It is this last element that is particularly likely to give rise to distress in nurses. It is an almost universal human reaction to be upset by seeing children in states of extreme unhappiness. The course offered by the ENB (course 603) is 46–49 weeks in length and its aim is to prepare experienced nurses for clinical and managerial roles in a service for disturbed children and adolescents. As part of the course there will be an introduction to many of the therapeutic approaches used with troubled children and their families, particularly family therapy. Participants in the course will also find themselves examining their own emotional responses in an effort to help them prepare for the difficulties of helping disturbed children and their families. Following the course, many participants will return to the clinical settings from which they came. These will not necessarily be mental health settings at all, but the new skills and knowledge of the specialist nursing in dealing with emotionally troubled children will help both her and her colleagues to examine emotional issues in general settings such as hospital wards, as well as in specialist facilities such as child guidance clinics, children's wards in psychiatric hospitals and community homes and schools.

CASE STUDY

Career development – Angie Hogg

Angie is an experienced staff nurse in a children's ward in a district general hospital. She has become increasingly worried by older children who are admitted to the ward following accidental and intentional overdoses. She is drawn towards them and wants to help but finds things difficult, both because the children typically stay for only a short time and because she does not feel she has the skills to talk to them about their problems in a way which will be helpful to them. Ultimately, she does not want to move into child and adolescent psychiatry, and in any case, she is not a Registered Mental Nurse, which would make promotion difficult. For Angie, the goal in her clinical work, is to possess sufficient skills to be able to counsel children in her current setting, and offer support to other staff and to parents concerning the emotional wellbeing of children, including those with specific emotional problems and those with anxieties associated with physical ill health.

EXERCISE

Use the nursing process to examine what Angie should do in deciding how to pursue her goal.

CONCLUSION

This chapter has presented just a selective picture of the wide range of specialities available within nursing. All post-basic courses should encourage the student to develop along the same lines, i.e. both professionally and personally. To ensure this, most ENB courses contain a common core of material, focusing on such issues as professional development and research skills. Furthermore, the courses should be personally challenging, encouraging the individual to seek out and adapt to changes in their clinical roles and ways of looking at those roles. A well-designed curriculum, which includes both a high level of up-to-date information and components of experiential learning which allow participants direct experience of their chosen specialities, will be challenging in this way whilst permitting the student sufficient safety to experiment with different ways of interacting as a specialist clinician with both clients and colleagues. The following personal perspective should really be about any well-organized post-basic course.

CASE STUDY

Post-basic education – a personal perspective
Colin Jacks is an 'E' grade staff nurse who completed a post-basic course six months ago. He both enjoyed and gained much from the experience, for example:

- an increased confidence, due Colin felt, to his improved understanding of the biological and behavioural sciences;
- an improvement in managing patient care due to an increase in research awareness related to a specific aspect of health care;
- an increase in job satisfaction through his ability to more effectively care for patients and their relatives in a variety of settings;
- a better understanding of the role of technology within health care;
- increased ability and confidence in teaching learners and less experienced qualified nurses and other professional colleagues.

EXERCISE

If after reading this chapter you are stimulated into looking, in more depth, at a career within a speciality, you are ready to carry out these two exercises.

1. Use the nursing process to guide your decision-making process. Use the case studies given in this chapter as templates.
2. Use the following steps to help in your decision making; the list of 'Useful Addresses' on page 171 may help you to access some of the information you need:
a) Investigate the available reading material relevant to the speciality.
b) Formulate some key questions you want to address.
c) If feasible, contact someone who is currently working within the relevant nursing field.
d) Write to the appropriate health/community trust personnel department to arrange an informal visit to a clinical area relevant to the speciality you wish to pursue.
e) Write to the appropriate educational institution requesting an informal visit with regard to the relevant post basic course that you may be interested in.

Further reading

English National Board for Nursing, Midwifery and Health Visiting Resource and Careers Department (1994) *Post Registration Courses – Opportunities for Continuing Education.* London: ENB.

Department of Health (1990) *Nursing in the Community* (HSC6). London: HMSO. (Sixth in a series published by the DOH – *Health Service Careers.*)

CHAPTER 9
The nurse in the community

Sandra Baulcomb

INTRODUCTION

Following first-level registration it is necessary for all nurses to undertake a period of consolidation in which the course of education they have just completed is put into practice. This may be compared with having driving lessons and then passing your test – most people say that the period *after* passing the test is the time when they learn to drive. Similarly for nurses, gaining experience in a nursing field is important to enable expertise to be developed, skills to be enhanced and a level of competence to be achieved.

After this period of consolidation, nurses may desire to progress as a nurse in a specialist field, and community nursing is a popular choice. The 'community', for the purpose of this chapter, is any setting where people go about their normal daily routines; it is where people live, go to school, go to work, play sports and take part in hobbies, recreation and their social life. It is within this complex network that community nurses practise. This requires an intimate knowledge of the community, its people, and the agencies which can provide help and support to the people. It is difficult to define the boundaries of a community nurse's role, but we shall try to do so later in this chapter, using three examples.

Because of recent changes in government policy there has been an increase in emphasis in providing care away from hospital settings to local communities, involving not only primary medical health care but also health prevention and health education. A team approach to care is widely recognized as an effective way of providing care across a range of activities in a co-ordinated and collaborative manner.[1]

EDUCATION AND TRAINING

The UKCC published a report in March 1994, setting out the future of nursing in the community and creating a new and unified discipline called 'Community Health Care Nursing'. This new discipline will 'reflect care skills required of all community nursing practitioners as well as additional specialist skills required for discrete areas of practice'.[2]

As part of this initiative, courses for preparation of community health care nurses will be at undergraduate level (level 3) and not be less than an academic year in length, although with Credit Accumulation and Transfer Systems (CATS) and Accreditation of Prior Experiential Learning (APEL) in operation individuals may find that through exemption, courses may be shorter.

Specialist modules will build on a common core and relate to specific areas of practice. The community health care nursing specialists of the future are as follows (in brackets is the term or description of the role as it has traditionally or historically been known):

- General Practice Nursing (Practice Nursing)
- Community Mental Health Nursing (Community Psychiatric Nursing)
- Community Mental Handicap Nursing (Community Nurse Mental Handicap)
- Community Children's Nursing (Community Paediatric)
- Public Health Nursing (Health Visiting)
- Occupational Health Nursing
- Nursing in the Home (District Nursing)
- School Nursing

The remainder of this chapter will look in more detail at the roles of practice nursing, health visiting and district nursing. Community psychiatric nursing and community nursing mental handicap are dealt with elsewhere in this book, as part of the chapters dealing with mental health and learning disabilities nursing. There is rather more blurring of roles between community and hospital practice in these fields than in the areas discussed below. Community paediatric nursing at the present time has an approach which is modelled on 'outreach' from hospitals rather than being a discrete area of community nursing practice. Community paediatric nurses are nurses who hold the Registered Sick Children's Nurse (RSCN) qualification and have not necessarily undertaken a community nursing preparation.

PRACTICE NURSING (GENERAL PRACTICE NURSING)

A practice nurse (PN) is usually a first-level Registered Nurse who is employed by a general practitioner to work within the general practice setting. Nurses have been working alongside doctors for quite some time, it being a rather ad hoc affair until 1966 with the emergence of the Family Doctors Charter, which allowed 70 per cent of salary costs to be reimbursed by the employing GP from the Family Practitioner Committee. In recent times the 1990 General Practitioner Contract[3] has been the single most important piece of legislation which has influenced the role of the practice nurse.

Following the implementation of the GP contract the work of the practice nurse became more diverse, moving away from task orientated treatment room work to a more holistic approach with health promotion and health education as the key. The treatment room function of the practice nurse, however, is important as this allows ambulant clients access to the nurse at times of appointment which are more convenient for the individual. The current role of the practice nurse can be shown as follows:

Role/Activity	Examples
Assessment	of the health needs of the practice population through practice profiling; of individual patient/client needs using a systematic approach; of own learning needs through personal profiling.
Planning	of goals and outcomes for the practice population based on health needs assessment; of goals and intervention for individual patients and clients; of courses to attend for professional updating.
Implementation	of plans of care for practice population and individual patients/clients; of skilled nursing intervention using appropriate interpersonal and communication skills.

Evaluation	of care given to practice population as a whole and individual patients and clients; comparison of actual outcomes with expected outcomes; of overall health gains and targets achieved in the practice.
Teaching	patients and clients about their illnesses and problems; skills to patients and clients to assist them in managing their problems themselves; health education activities in group and one-to-one situations; other nurses and professionals in the team.
Counselling	individuals with stress and anxiety within the nurse's sphere of competence; colleagues and the 'worried well' about concerns they may have; providing information.
Management	of time; of resources; of budgets as appropriate; of other nurses in the team; delegation of duties to others as appropriate.
Administration	record keeping; formulation of protocols and standards for practice; stock control; audit and quality control; formulation of contracts/purchasing agreements.
Technological	care and management of equipment; computer data storage and retrieval; safety in the work environment; use of minor surgical procedures; application of research.
Clinical	own professional updating; knowledge of disease processes; knowledge of treatments, drug protocols and interactions; application of research findings.

The practice nurse will be involved in a wide range of nursing activities, many of which allow the individual to extend her scope of practice well beyond traditional nursing roles. A large proportion of time is spent in health promotion activities and management of chronic disease. With the continued emphasis on community care and general practice in the future, the practice nurse role has great potential for nurses who wish to progress in this field

HEALTH VISITING (PUBLIC HEALTH NURSING)

The origins of health visiting lie in the period in which reforms of sanitary conditions were beginning to improve the general health of the population. In 1851 in Manchester, a Sanitary Association was formed, followed ten years later by the Ladies' Sanitary Association, to teach health to mothers. The effect of these organizations was at best inconclusive, so 'Respectable Women' were employed to go from home to home giving advice and help. These women volunteers became known as health visitors and, as the importance of their work in lowering the infant mortality rate became recognized, they were incorporated under the direction of the medical officer of health and their salary was paid by the local authority.

At this time, health visiting was seen as a separate profession from nursing as the health visitor's role was giving advice and educating the whole family, and with the continuing need to reduce the infant mortality rate, a statutory provision for health visiting was made. Along with this came the stipulation that health visitors must have either some medical, nursing or midwifery training before embarking on a course of health visitor training. Although health visitors see their work as concerning the whole family, a good deal of their time is spent in dealing with the needs of mothers and young children.

Over time developments and changes in health and social care have moulded the health visitor into the role occupied today. Health visitors are first-level registered nurses who have undertaken a further year of post-registration education in higher education at diploma or degree level to prepare them for the health visitor role. Health visitors are usually based in primary health care teams and are attached to a general practitioner group practice. The panel of patients who are registered with the group practice then become the potential caseload for the health visitor. These patients may be spread over a wide geographical area with several miles between each residence. Health visitors may also work in a geographical area or 'patch' which is defined by particular boundaries, the size of the patch usually relating to the number of people living in the area and the families within the patch becoming the potential caseload for the health visitor. Although the patch may be much more compact than a group attachment, the health visitor may have many more GPs to relate to.

Although health visitors have to be trained nurses before they can take up health visitor training, in reality little of their time is spent nursing in a clinical context. The main focus of health visitor activity is the promotion of health and prevention of ill health. To clarify what this means in practice, the Council for Education and Training of Health Visitors in 1977 reported on the findings of a working party:

> The professional practice of Health Visiting consists of planned activities aimed at the promotion of health and the prevention of ill health. It thereby contributes substantially to individual and social well being by focusing attention at various times on either an individual, a social group or community.4

From this report came the principles on which health visiting is based:

• The search for health needs.
• The stimulation of an awareness of health needs.
• Influence on policies affecting health.
• The facilitation of health enhancing activities.

The health visitor can achieve her aims through a combination of visiting individuals in their own homes and working with groups of people. On a one-to-one basis, much of the health visitor's time will be spent on home visits, where she can give complete attention to the family addressing their particular needs, for example helping a vulnerable parent develop self-esteem and parenting skills.

It is not appropriate to see some people as a member of a group, since they may not feel comfortable in this type of situation. Group work does, however, have its advantages and the health visitor may be able to achieve more through a group than working with individuals (e.g. a support group for carers of very dependent relatives, stress management workshops, practical demonstrations for parentcraft, making up an artificial feed). Group work can bring together people with similar needs and problems who may otherwise have felt isolated, and this may help boost confidence and develop skills. In reality, the health visitor will probably work with a combination of both these approaches in order to meet the needs of the families on the caseload, depending on local policies and approaches to management.

In addition to home visiting, the health visitor will also conduct clinic-based activities which maintain contact with families in between scheduled home visits. Such clinics may be child health clinics or well baby clinics, where the health visitor will give advice on any manner of issues such as feeding, weaning, sleep disturbance. Babies are assessed for normal patterns of development and any delay in development which may be detected. A doctor is often present at these clinics to provide a medical opinion and vaccination and immunization facilities.

Some health visitors may specialize and devote most of their time to particular client groups, for example elderly people, physically handicapped children, people with diabetes, or child protection. These health visitors will have undertaken the same broad-based education as generalist health visitors, but have developed a deeper, narrower remit, usually undertaking further training in their specialist area. Specialist health visitors are usually employed in addition to generalist health visitors.

EXERCISE

Compare and contrast the role of the generalist health visitor with the specialist health visitor. What do you believe are the advantages and disadvantages of each of these roles?

DISTRICT NURSING (NURSING IN THE HOME)

Modern-day district nursing in England began in Liverpool in 1859 through the initiative of a wealthy philanthropist, William Rathbone, whose wife died of tuberculosis. During her illness, a nurse, Mary Robinson, had been employed to care for her. After his wife's death William extended her contract for three months, so that she could work with the sick poor in Liverpool. Mary was soon overwhelmed as there was so much to do, and William was unable to find the calibre of nurse he wished to employ. After consulting with Florence Nightingale and following her advice, William founded a school of nursing, which was soon training nurses to work in people's homes and with the sick poor in the community. To allow the organization of the workload, a system was developed whereby the city was divided into 18 districts, hence the term district nursing.

District nurses are first-level Registered Nurses who have undertaken a further year of post-registration education in higher education at diploma or degree level to prepare them for their role. Like health visitors, district nurses are part of the primary health care team. By contrast, however, the district nurse usually works in a team of other community nurses, such as staff nurses, enrolled nurses and nursing auxiliaries (care assistants). The district nurse is the leader of the team of nurses and therefore has a major role to play in its management.

The district nurse works mainly in people's homes or wherever they may be living outside a hospital environment, including residential homes and hostels. She may also see patients in clinic settings and GPs' surgeries, if this enhances the care the patient will receive. As with the practice nurse, clinic- and surgery-based sessions may be more convenient for patients who are able to be out and about.

The district nurse will manage a caseload of patients, who are referred to her in a variety of ways. 44 per cent of referrals come from doctors, whilst 40 per cent are likely to be initiated by patients themselves. Other sources are hospital discharges and referrals from other primary health care team members (e.g. the health visitor). Patients who are referred usually have an existing health problem and will benefit from nursing intervention within the home. Examples of clients requiring district nursing care include:

- a 75-year-old woman with diabetes mellitus who needs assistance administering her insulin injection because her eyesight is failing;
- a 45-year-old man who has been discharged from hospital following an operation for ruptured appendix and now needs his wound dressing;
- a 65-year-old woman who is very immobile and in a lot of pain because of rheumatoid arthritis and needs assistance with washing and dressing every day;
- a 35-year-old man who has a brain tumour and is in the terminal stage of his life.

The 45-year-old man with the ruptured appendix may be classed as an acute case, as it would be expected that he would make a full recovery. By contrast, the other cases are classed as chronic, long-term conditions, which cannot be cured and will deteriorate over time, requiring more intervention from the health and social services. This second classification makes up the majority of the patients on a district nurse's caseload. Many of the patients are older and may not have anyone close by who can assist in their care.

It is the district nurse's responsibility to ensure that each patient who is on the caseload receives comprehensive and continuous care to meet their needs. The district nurse, for most of her day, is working alone and unsupervized. It is therefore most important that the standard of care she gives is the of highest possible quality, and the nurse must accept that she is personally accountable for the care given. The District Nurse Association UK has identified the following demands which are made on the district nurse in fulfilling her professional responsibilities towards patients and their carers:

a) *Initial assessment:* the district nurse will carry out the initial assessment when the patient is referred; this forms the basis on which nursing care is planned and care is prescribed. Care may then be delegated to other nurses in the team.

b) *Reassessment:* this takes place following evaluation of care to establish if outcomes and goals have been achieved, the effectiveness of the nurse's performance and the system of care adopted.

c) *Monitoring quality of care:* a skill which requires development and relies on the district nurse keeping reliable and accurate records. The use of information technology is increasingly important.

d) *Leadership:* providing leadership for the team includes providing motivation and opportunities for staff development to ensure the team are up to date in their practice.

e) *Delegation* of care to team members involves taking into account their individual abilities and areas of expertise. Supervision and monitoring of the team's performance is part of this role.

f) *Referral to other agencies* who have a part to play in the care of patients and families requires the district nurse to have an extensive knowledge of the local community, the statutory and voluntary agencies available, and skills to develop appropriate networks.

g) *Recognition of the importance of research* in informing district nursing practice.

h) *Analysis of the caseload* to reveal data that can form the basis of health needs assessment for the local community, to target areas of need and to facilitate effective use of available resources.

A final responsibility or demand made on the district nurse is the ability to teach and inform patients and their carers so they can also have a part to play either in their own care or in helping to care for a relative. Teaching may include safe lifting techniques, transferring from bed to wheelchair and even very technical procedures such as changing indwelling urinary catheters. As the district nurse is only

present in the patient's home for a relatively short time it is important that she is able to teach others so that care can continue.

District nurses can develop and extend the scope of their practice[5]
in order to provide comprehensive care. This may include taking
blood samples, ear syringing, setting up continuous drug delivery
systems, maintenance of intravenous infusions, caring for patients
on respirators and much more. The latest, and some believe most
important, development to date is the ability of district nurses (and
health visitors) to prescribe certain drugs, dressings and appliances
from a limited nurses' formulary.

CONCLUSION

This chapter has looked briefly at the nurse in the community, using
the three examples of the practice nurse, health visitor and district
nurse to illustrate the wide variety of nursing activity which is
undertaken. There is great scope for nurses who would like to practise in an alternative environment to the hospital which, though
being an essential part of our health care system, will see less emphasis placed in future. The community and primary health care arenas
will be the focus for much of the activity which takes place, so I
encourage any nurse with an interest to explore the possibilities
offered by nursing in the community.

EXERCISE

1. If you want to consider nursing in the community, think
    about the range of activities performed, and in particular
    examine the amount of additional responsibility involved
    in working in the community. Consider how you currently
    respond to responsibility and try to get a feeling for the
    effect an increase in this responsibility will have on you.
2. Molly Brown, the 65-year-old lady with rheumatoid
    arthritis referred to earlier is considerably disabled as a
    result of her condition. She is in severe pain; she can
    walk very slowly with the help of two people; eating and
    drinking is slow and laborious. In what ways could the
    district nursing team help to improve Molly's quality of
    life?

Further Reading

Robertson, C. (1991) *Health Visiting in Practice* (2nd Ed) Edinburgh. Churchill Livingstone.

Notes

1. DHSS (1986) *Neighbourhood Nursing. A Focus for Care.* (Cumberlege Report). London: HMSO.
2. UKCC (1994) *The Future of Professional Practice – the Councils Standards for Education and practice following Registration,* 13. London: UKCC .
3. DOH (1990) *The GP Contract.* London: HMSO.
4. CETHV (1977) *An Investigation into the Principles of Health Visiting.* London: CETHV.
5. UKCC (1992) *The Scope of Professional Practice.* London: UKCC.

CHAPTER 10
The nurse as a manager

David Justham

INTRODUCTION

Nurses look after patients and their families in a range of settings, including hospital, in the community, and in the general practitioner's surgery. Many of these providers of health care are large organizations, employing sometimes thousands of staff, which need to be managed well if they are going to be effective in meeting the care needs of patients.

There are several levels of management. *First line managers* are responsible for staff who are delivering care, for example the ward sister, district nurse, or practice nurse manager); next are *middle managers* who have responsibilities for a number of first line managers: the senior nurse manager in a clinical directorate within a hospital is a good example. At the most senior level within an organization are those managers who seek to ensure that the whole organization is working well, that there is co-ordination between different departments, and that the organization is able to respond to changes in clinical practice and patterns of disease; the nurse adviser to an NHS Trust operates at this level. Even within the different levels of management, a wide range of managerial jobs exists, in which nurses can make a valuable, indeed essential, contribution.

In this chapter I will introduce you to some of the areas to reflect upon in deciding whether you want to develop a career in management, to some of the situations in which nurses perform management roles, and refer to the experiences which face many people who take on such roles for the first time. Just as nurses need specific training in order to work in particular areas of nursing, so too the training needs of managers will be addressed.

WHAT MANAGERS DO

Management is an exciting and challenging area in which to work, carrying responsibility for ensuring that the work of the organization is achieved. In nursing terms, managers co-ordinate resources, making sure there is enough staff and equipment to give good patient care. They plan for the future, so that changing patterns of health care are met with appropriately skilled and able staff. Managers are engaged in leading staff, and participating in the corporate life of the organization so that all aspects of the service are working to the same purpose – the delivery of health care.

There are many different books that describe what managers do (a list of key texts is provided at the end of this chapter), and you will find alternative accounts describing the manager's job. One such author is Mintzberg[1] who has described 10 roles for the manager:

Inter-personal roles: Figurehead; Leader; Liaison.
Informational roles: Monitor; Disseminator; Spokesman.
Decisional roles: Entrepreneur; Disturbance Handler; Resource Allocator; Negotiator.

Inter-personal roles

Inter-personal roles are those to do with leading your team. At various times this will require you to be a figurehead – to be the person who 'carries the can' when things don't go to plan, or who is the central point of reference within the team. The ward sister or charge nurse is seen as a figurehead: when strangers arrive on the ward they will ask 'Is Sister on duty?' She becomes the person to whom everyone refers. Research undertaken in the 1970s[2] showed that, on a typical morning, a ward sister can expect to be in conversation with different people an average of twenty times per hour (excluding conversations with patients and their relatives, or any held using the telephone).

Managers are also leaders. They are required to set the standards to which their staff must work and to take action to ensure that the standards are maintained. They lead by example, by motivating staff and by bringing together the right mix of resources to ensure the task of caring is completed successfully. The manager must be capable of liaising with others: her staff expect this. It is necessary from time to time to talk to other departmental heads about co-ordination of services. For example, when a new service is being planned which requires additional clinic space, the manager will need to liaise with the clinic manager about the availability of space, and the days and times in the week when the space is available.

Leaders in nursing need to recognize their own responsibilities under the UKCC's Code of Conduct, as well as recognizing the implications of the Code for those they lead.

Informational roles

Informational roles are about communication, which is vital for effective management. The monitoring role refers to the need to gather and review information. Managing a budget requires financial information, managing staff workload requires information about patient dependency and activity levels. Making sure the service meets customer needs calls for information about customer satisfaction. Without such information, the manager cannot be in control, nor can she be able to plan the future work programme, or know how much money is available to buy new equipment. Dissemination involves you in passing on information. If staff do not know what is happening they become suspicious and demotivated. Managers need to hand on information. It is no good expecting staff to attend a fire lecture if they don't know it is taking place! Likewise, if other managers do not know what your plans are there will be confusion and poor co-ordination. There are times when you need to be the spokeswoman for your team, in ways which echo the role of figurehead.

Decisional roles

Making decisions is the area of managerial work which is often the most challenging. This is particularly so where there are limited resources, and the manager must decide between two or more competing priorities. Staff, and indeed representatives of the public, do not always appreciate these limitations. For example, a senior nurse may have to decide between allowing one nurse to attend a costly post-basic course (which could use the majority of the training budget for the year), or using the money to enable more staff to attend other courses. Both actions would benefit the team as a whole but whatever the decision, someone will be disappointed. The manager must implement her decision, and be able explain reasonably why the particular choice was made. In this context, we see that the manager is also a resource allocator. When the workload is high across the four wards which a senior nurse may manage and resources are limited, where does she allocate the one agency nurse or bank nurse who has been brought in for the shift? From time to time, things do not go according to plan. For many, this is the challenge of management, *making it happen*, despite the difficulties that occur along the way.

Mintzberg's roles apply whatever the level of management, although they do not all apply with equal weight in each job. Some jobs emphasize more the informational roles, whereas others require the decisional roles to take prominence. The roles apply to nurses as managers just as much as they apply to any manager. Many managers will tell you that their work is demanding, they have to be able to handle pressure and work to deadlines. In order to get the job done they will need to delegate, which is one aspect of being able to manage time effectively. Inter-personal skills are paramount; managers spend a lot of time in meetings, whether in committees or on a one-to-one basis, taking and making telephone calls, interviewing for new staff and listening to existing staff. What, then, are the skills needed to perform these roles and tasks effectively?

SKILLS NEEDED TO MANAGE

Nurses are at an advantage over many managers in that their training involves development of inter-personal skills. Nurses are used to listening to and talking with patients, their families, friends and carers: inter-personal skills used in management are based on the same principles. Nurses tend to be skilled in aspects of non-verbal communication, and in handling the mechanics of a conversation, like starting and finishing an interview. The nurse who moves into management will need to develop these skills further, because even though the principles may be similar, interviewing for new staff is quite a different experience from interviewing a new patient.

Managers have to cope with pressure. These pressures may be to do with timescale – everybody wants the job done yesterday! This is more apparent these days, partly due to the general speed of modern society, and partly due to the changing nature of the health services, with constantly new and improved technologies or government policies driving the pace of change. Pressure also comes from workload. Demands are made on managers by their senior manager to meet particular objectives or supply information. Expectations are placed on managers by staff who are looking to them to resolve their difficulties in delivering care. The need to get answers to questions, to plan for co-ordination of services, calls for liaison with others. For example, a nurse manager responsible for introducing a home support service for terminally ill patients would need to liaise with managers of district nurses, the local hospice, GPs, and hospitals.

Particular pressures face the new manager and these are discussed below. Pressure can lead to stress, and managers need to be able to handle stress. Courses on stress management are commonplace these days. Other techniques can also help – compartmentalizing is used to separate the work into manageable portions. This is best seen in managers going on 'Away Days' – that is, getting away from the office for a period to complete work on a particular issue.

Time management is another much-needed skill. Whether we are managers or not, many of us do not get the best from the time available. Managers need to be able to organize their time effectively if they are to keep their desk clear and to keep on top of their work. Diary management is a crucial feature in this area. The following case study shows a typical day for a senior nurse, with a series of meetings, lists of telephone calls to make and people to see. Secretaries or personal assistants help managers enormously by controlling the access of others to them.

CASE STUDY

A day in the life of a nurse manager
8.30 a.m. Attend daily multidisciplinary ward meeting to discuss patient progress. Afterwards meet each member of staff briefly, and assess how they see the day progressing, and the likely resource requirements for which they may need help.
9.00 a.m. In office, making and receiving telephone calls, and dealing with post. Dictation with secretary.
9.30 a.m. Bereavement counselling for relatives of Mrs ——.

10.15 a.m. Discussion with colleagues, over coffee, concerning duties to be allocated to new volunteers.
11.00 a.m. Visit the ward and day care unit to assess how staff are coping, and meet patients.
11.30 a.m. Staff appraisal interview with Sister ———.
12.30 p.m. Lunch.
1.00 p.m. Office work, planning for future changes, preparation for teaching session. Taking telephone calls from colleagues on aspects of care management.
2.30 p.m. Dealing with staff sickness, contacting 'bank' staff to provide additional manpower for the evening.
3.00 p.m. Teaching session on Bereavement Counselling to student nurses.
4.00 p.m. Meeting with General Manager to discuss budget issues.
4.30 p.m. Visit ward to ensure that arrangements for the evening and night-time care are satisfactory. Meet patients and identify that needs are being met.
5.00 p.m. Attend to unresolved issues, make further telephone calls, complete correspondence, and finalize paperwork on staff appraisal interview. Home.

(With acknowledgement to Penny McFaul.)

The art of delegation is a skill to be learnt. Nurses begin learning this when they lead a team for a shift, enabling the team to care for a number of patients effectively. Delegation enables others to work for you, since the job becomes too big if you try to do it all yourself. It serves at least two other functions: delegation enables the manager to prepare staff who may be looking to develop a career in management, and through the opportunity given, enables the member of staff to appreciate more the task of management; delegation also enables the manager to free time to address other issues. The skill in delegation is to delegate work which it is reasonable and appropriate for others to undertake. Never delegating will lead to work overload. Delegating inappropriately will lead you into difficulties very quickly.

Getting the job done through others will need the manager to be assertive. There will be times when staff do not see the reason for particular requests, or show reluctance to perform the duty requested. The skill of the manager is to be able to encourage the member of staff to accept the task without feeling pressurized into doing so. The manager needs to be assertive when dealing with colleagues; in meetings, for example, it may be necessary to stand your ground for the benefit of your team. The manager may need to argue for additional resources, or seek to maintain existing resources when cutbacks, or efficiency savings, are being sought. Assertiveness is a characteristic of the skilled negotiator. Negotiation is successful only when all parties involved feel that they have achieved their objectives. This is known as getting to a 'win-win' situation.

In addition to these skills you will bring others to your work as a manager. For instance, you will have technical skills related to nursing. It is useful to reflect on these and how they are used. The systematic approach you probably adopt when looking after the individual patient goes through the stages of assessing care needs, deciding on the care needs, planning how to meet those care needs, implementing the plan of care, and reviewing the effect of the care given. This skill lends itself easily to the rational approach to introducing change (for example, a new way of working). The manager will assess the situation, collecting together whatever information is available or undertaking some research; she will then decide, on the basis of the information, what is the best option for change. The next stage is to prepare a plan for implementation which will include informing the people affected by the proposed change, anticipating any additional training which they may need, and bidding for resources. Once the plan is agreed, the next stage is to implement the new working system. There may be initial teething problems, but once these have been resolved there will be a review of the plan and its implementation to assess if the change in practice has achieved the objectives intended.

Another skill is that of being able to conceptualize – this is the ability to identify the significant elements in a given situation, a skill most nurses have. They are able, for example, to assess clinical emergencies, to understand the implications for patients, and to initiate the necessary response.

Managers need 'political' skills, that is the ability to handle the system, to know the formal channels of communication, and to identify where the power and authority lie within an organization. Nurses often become adept in this area in order to achieve the best for their patients. Using these abilities in the managerial context ensures that the staff who report to you are more likely to get the resources and support they need.

TYPES OF MANAGEMENT JOBS

The nurse who is looking to management as a career should be aware that there is not only a need for nurses to manage nurses and nursing, but an important place for nurses in other managerial roles too. Throughout the health service nurses can be found in all aspects and levels of management. Some management posts held by nurses include:

Within NHS purchasing:
  Chief executives of health authorities or purchasing commissions
  Directors of contracting and commissioning
  Directors of quality assurance
  Nurse advisers to health authorities or purchasing commissions
  Planning managers or quality assurance managers

Within NHS providers:
  Chief executives of NHS Trusts
  Directors of contracting
  Directors of personnel
  Directors of nursing and quality assurance
  Quality assurance managers
  Information managers
  Business managers
  Senior nurse managers
  Ward managers or caseload managers

Within local authority social service departments:
  Care managers (in respect to care management arrangements following the introduction of 'Caring for People')

Voluntary and private sector:
  Managers of nursing homes
  Nurses in charge of nursing homes
  Home leaders
  Shift managers

This list shows some of the variety of jobs available in management. Posts in *quality assurance* are frequently held by nurses. Nurses are the one professional group who can claim to be with patients 24 hours a day. They serve as advocates for the patient, and have an all-round perspective of the care needs of the patient. To this end, they are well placed to manage the quality assurance activities of health care organizations. This age of consumerism, and the need to demonstrate that a quality service is being delivered, calls for skilled quality assurance managers.

Another growth area is that of *health care purchasing*. The reforms of the NHS have resulted in health authorities and GP fund holders becoming purchasers of health care. Effective purchasing requires good contracts which clearly identify what the purchaser wishes the provider of health care to do. Purchasing managers who have clinical backgrounds are best placed to buy health care, and this requires nurses to be at the forefront in contract management.

Business management is another area calling for special comment. Within health care organizations there are those who manage the interface with purchasers of health care. In many this responsibility rests with the business manager, who frequently works within a clinical directorate alongside a senior nurse manager. The need to ensure management efficiency is resulting in the role of the business manager being merged with that of the senior nurse manager in many instances. Such posts provide exciting challenges for nurses.

The career structure in nurse management has changed significantly in recent years. The traditional career ladder, solely concerned with managing nursing (so-called 'functional management') has largely disappeared. Nor is it possible to point to a pay scale solely for nurse managers; indeed these days nurses in management positions will more often than not be paid on a scale common to their non-nursing managerial colleagues. Managers are judged on their performance in meeting particular objectives within given timescales. These objectives will be set by their line manager and are almost certainly a reflection of the targets which the line managers have been set by their own superiors. In the NHS, performance-related pay may be a part of the employment package, the levels of pay being determined in relation to how successful the manager has been in achieving and surpassing short-, medium- and long-term objectives. In some situations, this system of bonus reward is being replaced by a team bonus which recognizes the contribution made by a managerial team as a whole, because of the interdependence one member has on another in achieving a desired outcome. Within a clinical directorate in a large acute hospital, the clinical director, senior nurse manager and business manager may share a team bonus.

Entry to a management career normally begins with an appointment to a first line manager post. Examples are the ward manager (the traditional ward sister or charge nurse role), or caseload manager in a community setting (whether as a district nurse, health visitor, community psychiatric nurse or community nurse for people with a learning disability), or as a practice nurse manager (found in large GP practices which employ several practice nurses). These first line posts present particular challenges because there is often a requirement for the manager to be clinically involved as well.

THE TRAINING NEEDS OF MANAGERS

You will find many managers who believe experience as a manager is the best training. This is like learning by trial and error, and does not lead, necessarily, to the best management practices. The view is changing, and today there are opportunities for management training. Many senior positions in management require managers to have formal qualifications in management. In health care organizations, these qualifications could be a certificate or diploma in managing health services, or a masters degree in business management. Increasingly, middle management positions require candidates to show evidence of formal training in management. Some useful addresses for information are shown at the end of this chapter.

In addition, your local college of further or higher education, or university will probably have a Department of Business Studies or Business School which would supply information. If your employer has a training department, contacting them may also be useful.

TAKING THE FIRST STEP

Deciding to pursue a career in management will lead to your first managerial post. Here are some issues to reflect on. Firstly, there is the *player-manager* syndrome. What the syndrome identifies is that sometimes managers prefer to return to the clinical area rather than address the issues facing them as a manager. This demonstrates some insecurity (which is natural in a new role) but can be counter-productive in providing leadership for staff, and in learning the art of delegation. It is not unusual to experience this, though some new managers think they are failing because of the dual role they seem to be leading. In essence the experience is one of letting go, of allowing others to do the work which you need to leave behind as a manager. Is it possible to be a caring nurse, yet at the same time be able to take tough managerial decisions, decisions which others may see as not in the best interests of patient care? I believe it is. As a full-time manager you will need to consider the best way to maintain clinical credibility. For example, you may want to make time to work in a clinical area. This may not be easy, and you might experience opposition from managerial colleagues. It is important to draw the distinction here from managerial posts which also *require* a clinical component. In these posts maintenance of the balance between management responsibilities and clinical duties is important.

The transition from one role to another can also cause stress. This may arise from role ambiguity (not being completely sure what the job is about), or from role conflict (becoming aware of the need to exert discipline on staff with whom you were previously a workmate). Most people accommodate well to the transition, though in the early days of the job, the new manager may question whether she has done the right thing.

In practical terms, taking the first step towards management requires you to talk with those who are in first line manager posts. Find out directly what it is like. Many managers enjoy the challenges of being able to influence a wider area of work than the limited sphere they were involved in previously. They enjoy the freedom to make decisions, and the ability to control budgets, to appoint staff, and to influence others. Talk to your line managers about your hopes and aspirations for the future; they may be able to give you developmental opportunities like managing a project or being an 'acting' ward manager for a period if a colleague should be on long-term sickleave, or before a vacancy is filled. Such 'acting' opportunities allow you the experience of taking charge for real, with the option to return to your normal job at the end of the period. Take time to find out about the management training courses which may be suitable for you.

EXERCISE

1. Reflect on the following:
   a) Why do I want to be a manager?
   b) Do I believe I can make a contribution to patient care by being a manager?
   c) Which of Mintzberg's roles excite me?
   d) Which of these roles do I already have experience in – perhaps through non-work activities?
   e) Which do I need to develop?

2. Talk to others:
   a) Your line managers – find out from them what their experience of management has been like, and what opportunities might be available to you.
   b) Other managers you know, within or outside health care, and find out about their jobs.
3. Get information on training opportunities for the types of management job to which you are attracted.
4. If you decide on a management career, plan for a move to a first line management post, and where you would like to be in five years' time.

Addresses for information about management training

The Institute of Health Service Management, 39 Chalton Street, London NW11 1JD.

The Open Business School, The Open University, Walton Hall, Milton Keynes MK7 6AA.

The National Health Service Training Directorate, St Bartholomews Court, 18 Christmas Street, Bristol BS1 5BT.

Further reading

General texts
Drucker, P. (1980) *Management*. London: Pan.
Handy, C. (1993) *Understanding Organizations*. Harmondsworth: Penguin.
Peters, T. J., and Waterman, R. H. (1982) *In Search of Excellence*. London: Harper & Row.
Stewart, R. (1970) *The Reality of Management*. London: Pan.

Nursing texts
Dodwell, M., and Lathlean, J. (Eds) (1989) *Management & Professional Development for Nurses*. London: Harper & Row.
Matthews, A. (1982) *In Charge of the Ward*. Oxford: Blackwell Scientific.

Macleod Nicol, N., and Walker, S. (1991) *Basic Management for Staff Nurses*. London: Chapman Hall.
Stewart, R. (1989) *Leading in the NHS: A Practical Guide*. London: Macmillan.

Notes

1. Mintzberg, H. (1973) *The Nature of Managerial Work*. London: Harper and Row.
2. Lelean, S. R. (1973) *Ready for Report Nurse?* London: Royal College of Nursing.

CHAPTER 11
The nurse as a teacher

Peter Birchenall

INTRODUCTION

From the outset of a nurse's training there is an emphasis on health rather than illness. Good physical and mental health is an essential prerequisite to a normal life, and nurses are therefore educated to view illness and disability as an impediment to a healthy existence. The role of the nurse and other health care workers is to work in partnership with each other and with the patient in removing or reducing the effect of this impediment. Nursing is not preoccupied with a disease orientation, but sees the individual as having personal responsibility for maintaining his own health. In the case of young children or profoundly disabled people this responsibility passes to parents, guardians, and informal carers. Patient education is aimed at empowering people to recognize the part they can play in caring for themselves and others in health and illness, through an analysis of their lifestyles, and making changes or adjustments where necessary. In this way, all nursing is about patient education, and some of this chapter will examine how the nurse, in the course of her clinical role, undertakes patient education of this kind. However, some nurses expand the educational component of their job greatly, by choosing to concentrate, for example, on health education and promotion, or on the professional and academic education of nurses and other health professionals. This chapter deals with both these aspects of nursing as education, and also contains information and examples both to help you to decide whether you wish to take this direction in your nursing career and to show you some of the practicalities involved.

PATIENT EDUCATION

Can you envisage an aspect of your own health which you would appreciate knowing more about? If the answer is 'Yes', have you thought about asking your local practice nurse or health visitor to advise you? Whenever a nurse responds to such a request for information, she is acting as an educator.

Historically, the hierarchical structure within hospitals created a situation which demanded unchallenged compliance by patients to doctor's orders. Those patients who did not comply with the doctor's instructions, or questioned a certain treatment regime would be labelled as unco-operative, and may have become quite unpopular. This approach to hospital care has largely given way to a more informed, patient-centred approach to care planning, where the patient is included every step of the way. The more the balance has shifted towards the notion of informed, involved patients, the greater has been the increase in the need for good educational skills amongst clinical nurses, who are typically at the forefront of the endeavour to put across to patients the need to co-operate with clinicians in dealing with their difficulties.

The old saying 'prevention is better than cure' makes a lot of sense, but unfortunately some people follow a lifestyle that can, and often does, affect their health in a negative fashion. For example, disorders of health related to tobacco products, obesity, stress, excess alcohol consumption and preventable accidents account for many admissions and readmissions to hospital. Take as a case in point someone who smokes excessively and is admitted to hospital with severe chest problems. The commonsense thing for that person to do would be to cut down on cigarettes or give up smoking altogether. Creating an awareness of the harm that can accrue from a continuation of smoking would be an essential part of the nursing care plan for this individual. The nurse would be applying her knowledge and expertise as a teacher in an effort to improve her patient's chance of a full recovery.

A substantial part of a nurse's daily work is teaching patients or clients how to look after themselves. This may vary from simple advice on smoking, diet or exercise to more complicated activities associated with the specialized nature of an individual patient's care.

Examples, such as self-injection of insulin or teaching a stroke victim how to dress himself, are quite common. From my own experience I can recall helping an elderly man who had suffered paralysis down one side of his body, resulting in partial loss of speech, to communicate his needs. This was achieved by making a cardboard clock face upon which words such as 'toilet', 'drink', 'rest', and 'sit up' were clearly written. A pointer was secured to the centre of this simple structure and the patient was able to use his unaffected hand to indicate his immediate need by positioning the pointer appropriately.

EXERCISE

Can you think of any other situation where a patient or client would possibly require some help in learning or re-learning a daily living activity, and how this may be achieved by the nurse?

Recent years have seen the advancement and growth of nursing knowledge into specialist activities such as palliative care, operating theatre nursing, diabetic care, coronary care, stoma care, and many others. As a result there has arisen a need for nurses to become highly skilled in the art of patient education. Teaching skills allied to nursing skills form the basis of effective care in many situations because a patient who is well informed becomes an active partner in his care.

Many patients receiving hospital care often find the length of stay to be quite short, even after major surgery. Therefore it becomes important for this partnership in care to continue following discharge from hospital. Follow-up care at home must be carried out effectively, consequently it becomes essential for the patient and his family to be aware of potential problems which may arise along the way to full recovery. Prior to discharge, clear guidance by hospital staff in the form of written advice, or simple verbal instruction, is part of the nurse's teaching function. There are many examples of well-designed educational materials, produced by nurses, which get the message across in uncomplicated, non-medical language. Innovative nurses now make use of audio and video tapes to provide an educational service for their patients, the latter often demonstrating how to carry out routine activities in a safe manner.

Continuation of care at home is the responsibility of community services, which include district nurses, health visitors and other more specialist carers, such as Macmillan nurses involved in the care of people with cancer. The nature of the work of these specialists in nursing in the community is determined by the needs of the patient, and can vary from carrying out routine procedures such as dressings and injections, to counselling, advising and instructing both the patient and informal carers on day-to-day care.

Caring does not cease in between visits, but carries on, following a plan agreed and discussed with the patient and her informal carer. Since the nurse cannot be with the person at all times, continuing care is the responsibility of the person and her family; thus patient/client education features prominently and is essential to the maintenance of care. Involvement is the key word, and through effective teaching the community nurse and health visitor can create a caring environment which remains supportive at all times. Teaching someone else how to perform some skill which we ourselves take for granted often requires a high level of understanding of that skill, of ourselves and the needs of others, so patient teaching of this kind is a challenging area.

People with mental health problems and those with forms of disability living at home will require nursing support which includes a properly directed teaching function. Community psychiatric nurses, for example, spend much of their time working with clients in a teaching capacity. Recovery from a mental health problem can be a slow process, and learning to readjust to everyday life demands a careful and well-planned approach by the nurse. Strategies are employed which enable the individual to meet and overcome problems along the way to recovery. Group work or one-to-one activities are used, with the nurse acting as facilitator. The skills of facilitation and communication are central to effective teaching, and can be found at the heart of mental health nursing. Community learning disability nurses also have a major teaching component to their role. Theirs is a job that promotes self-care and integration of people with learning disabilities into the community. They not only teach their clients, but also spend time educating members of the community about learning disabilities, as a means of dispelling myths and prejudices. See chapter 5 for further information and examples of the nurse's teaching role in this specialist field.

NURSE TEACHING

The student nurse as a teacher

As well as teaching patients, nurses also teach each other in the practice and theory of caring. During my own student days I can remember times when I discovered how to do something by asking another student who was more senior and experienced than myself. Often the instruction would be accompanied by up-to-the-minute theory gained from lectures or reading. This valuable form of teaching and learning is part of the 'hidden curriculum' of nurse education and its importance often goes unrecognized. Where it is recognized and included as part of the 'formal curriculum' there exists a rich vein of opportunity not only in teaching and learning, but also in promoting peer support and cohesion between students at different levels of the course.

Timetables can be co-ordinated to enable senior students to adopt the role of mentor in the clinical area. This happens in the undergraduate nursing degree course at Hull University where each 4th-year student is given responsibility for a maximum of two less experienced 1st-year students on one day each week over two academic terms. Together they carry out a series of predetermined basic caring activities such as bathing a patient, treatment of pressure areas, taking and recording temperature, pulse and respiration, and measuring and recording blood pressure. The senior students are prepared for this aspect of their role by following an assessed course in teaching and learning in clinical practice which contributes towards their overall final degree classification. The junior students follow a parallel course in the theory of that particular week's subject as preparation for the practical experience. In order to keep within the training requirements, academic and qualified ward staff maintain a discrete but careful watch over the arrangements, but problems are rare. The benefits outweigh any disadvantages, and both sets of students gain immeasurably from the relationship.

This process of peer mentorship helps the senior student to integrate teaching into her role, a process which will continue throughout her nursing career. Registered Nurses teach students and care assistants as part of their daily work, and in the more formal setting of a classroom students are taught by trained teachers who themselves are qualified nurses. There is also a specialist nurse called a lecturer/practitioner who works with students in both classroom and clinical areas, whilst maintaining a considerable clinical caseload and thereby acting as a role model of clinical excellence for learner nurses. These different teaching roles will now be considered further.

HOW NURSES LEARN TO TEACH

The governing body for nursing, midwifery and health visiting insists that at all times students are properly supervized and taught by appropriately trained people. Job descriptions for staff nurses and more senior nurses at clinical level contain a requirement to teach. Before a clinical area, either in hospital or the community, can become approved for nurse training there has to be evidence that it has the necessary resources to support students and provide them with a range of relevant experiences. This can only be achieved where sufficient members of the nursing staff are available for teaching purposes. Each student has to be attached to a personal mentor – a qualified nurse – whose role is to ensure that learning opportunities are provided and placement objectives are met. Mentorship is taken very seriously and people are trained in its skills and complexities. This training is usually carried out over two or three days and covers the basics of how to instruct students, including writing a teaching plan, creating a learning environment, and acquiring basic practical teaching skills.

Mentorship can be a rewarding experience for both student and mentor. It is encouraging when new skills come to fruition and a sense of achievement is realized. There are also the frustrations associated with students who make only slow progress, but mentors are prepared for this and with patience can sort out most difficulties. It is often more rewarding to know that one has helped the less gifted student to achieve her potential for success than to work with the very able student who has less need of direction and support to reach the same level of competence.

EXERCISE

Consult a dictionary and find the origin of the term 'mentor'. Now consider how the term's original meaning might be translated into the actions of the mentor in nursing. If you are already a qualified nurse and have acted as a mentor yourself, examine how your role corresponds to this original meaning of the word.

Qualified nurses who wish to concentrate more fully on teaching can follow one of several pathways. It is advisable to take a course of study approved by one or more of the statutory nursing boards for England, Wales, Scotland or Northern Ireland. These courses range from relatively short certificate of attendance programmes in teaching and assessing in clinical practice (such as the ENB 998), to full- or part-time courses leading to a diploma or honours degree in nursing education, and qualified nurse teacher status. Diploma courses for health care professional teachers are also offered to a wide range of qualified health professionals including nurses. These courses reflect a multidisciplinary approach to teacher preparation using a shared knowledge base, and in a similar way to the conventional routes, have to be approved by the statutory nursing body before the qualification is recognized. The precise location of the nearest course can be found by writing to the National Nursing Board of whichever part of the UK in which you live or work. These addresses are included at the end of this book (see pages 171, 172).

BECOMING A QUALIFIED TEACHER OF NURSES

Entry to a recognized teacher training course and subsequent recording of the qualification is not easy. The UKCC stipulate a number of strict conditions to be met before any application is considered:

- The applicant must be a Registered Nurse.
- The applicant must have recently completed at least three years post-registration experience, two years of which must be in the United Kingdom working where pre-registration students are allocated for experience.
- There are regulations governing part-time and nurse bank work which stipulate that periods of time under six months are not recognized for the purpose of experience.
- The applicant must be recommended by her senior manager as being a suitable person for nurse teacher preparation.
- The applicant must also meet the academic entry criteria laid down by the institution offering the course. It is likely that a degree will be the minimum entry qualification.
- The recording of any resulting qualification is at the discretion of the UKCC, and under normal circumstances the applicant will have occupied a funded place on an approved course.

- Applicants who have gained an approved qualification but do not meet the post-registration experience criteria generally have to seek specific advice from the UKCC. In certain circumstances it is possible to make up the experience and then work under the supervision of a qualified teacher for a stipulated period of time. Each case is viewed on its merits and unless a procedure has been agreed at the outset, it can be a prolonged and frustrating route to qualification.

THE LECTURER/PRACTITIONER

Resulting from the need to educate students rather than just train them, teachers of nurses spend much of their time in formal settings such as classrooms and lecture theatres. Their role is to give students the sound theoretical education so essential to modern nursing, particularly as effective care should be determined by the application of quality research. It is in the application of theory to practice where teaching is at its most potent, and the introduction of a teacher who also takes responsibility for a clinical caseload can be beneficial to students and patients. Caring and learning go together, but this is not simply a case of using an apprenticeship system in which learning is unstructured and many tasks of dubious educational value are performed by learners. The role of the lecturer/practitioner is to focus on active learning, giving students hands-on experience coupled with related theory. In short lecturer/practitioners ensure that students understand the 'what', 'how' and 'why' of nursing.

There is no recognized nationally approved preparation for this job at present, but courses do exist in some parts of the country, and a number attract regional funding. These courses have various names and it is not always clear if their purpose is to offer lecturer/practitioner training. Interested readers should direct enquiries to their regional nurse responsible for continuing education, or write direct to the university or college where the course is offered.

CONCLUSION

This chapter has touched upon some of the teaching activities carried out by nurses. It has not by any means described them all, because whatever caring situation nurses find themselves in whether it be a hospital ward, a patient's home, a prison hospital or a local GP surgery, it is likely they will be teaching something to someone. Teaching is an extension of the caring function, and one without the other would be unthinkable to most nurses, because health promotion and education represent vital elements of the nursing role. One of the great challenges for nurse education is to be able to keep pace with rapid change, whether this be in educational theory, nursing and medical technology and knowledge, or the role of the nurse within the health care system.

CHAPTER 12
The nurse as a researcher

Rachel Tucker

INTRODUCTION

For many, the practice of research is not usually associated with the practice of nursing. Indeed when people ask about what options are available within a nursing career, research is not an area that immediately springs to mind. It can be as new an interest to someone who is already a qualified nurse as it can be to someone who is considering entering the nursing profession. Many courses now involve research within their curriculum. However, its history is fairly short and so nurses often become interested or prioritize other specialities before research.

Research is not just about finding solutions to problems, though in its broadest sense it can be described as such. It is a systematic enquiry that uses scientific rules (that is, the research process) to seek conclusions in an unbiased and objective manner. It is therefore very important as it can aid the development of an individual's or a group's body of knowledge by means of the discovery of new facts or information.

So what do you feel about research? Perhaps you feel that research is too 'academic' and detached from patient contact, or perhaps you may even think of it as boring, or that you're the wrong sort of person to become a researcher. If you are uncertain about the type of qualities a nurse researcher needs, or even what sort of person becomes a nurse researcher, then try answering the following questions and see if they match your own personal characteristics:

- Do you have an inquisitive mind?
- Do you have an interest in improving patient care, promoting good health and preventing illness?
- Are you self-motivated?
- Do you have the ability to plan and co-ordinate your own work?
- Do you enjoy communicating with others?
- Do you have the ability to work on your own as well as within a team?

For those who may be about to embark on nurse training, you may feel that you do not have many of the above attributes. However, many potential nurses have such characteristics and you will find that these will be developed during your nurse education. For those who are already qualified nurses, you may recognize that often the skills associated with being a proficient nurse researcher are the same as those associated with being a proficient nurse.

THE NURSE AS A CONSUMER AND INITIATOR OF RESEARCH

The nurse is in the best position for identifying potential problems relating to patient care. She is often the one that spends the most time with patients by the bedside and therefore can frequently ascertain whether a particular procedure, treatment or attitude is effective or ineffective. In the past, nursing practice was more reliant on tradition or intuition rather than on evidence, and research remained a relatively new area. Today in nursing it is recognized as the means of providing scientifically established knowledge to improve and develop patient care, to defend specific nursing activities and to secure professional status for nursing.

Nurses, however, are occasionally apprehensive about their role as researchers, and may harbour negative attitudes and expectations of research. This will be particularly apparent if the experience of education has not promoted an enquiring mind through the reading of research reports and the discussion of findings. The practice of research is also often accused of alienating sections of the nursing profession. The fact that there are many definitions of research does little to aid the development of a novice or potential nurse researcher. Indeed, it is not surprising that such a multitude of definitions confuses and deters nurses before they even begin to contemplate other procedures relating to the research process.

A good education and knowledge-base of research is essential to promote both research awareness and a valid background for clinical practice. Even if all individuals do not become fully involved within research, such experience can only lead to a greater understanding and utilization of research findings within clinical practice, and will therefore help to improve patient care.

Nurses are in an excellent position to become efficient consumers of research. Nurses who are aware of the most recent knowledge relating to their particular area of practice will not only improve the care of individual patients and clients, but will also improve the reputation of the profession. Formerly, nurses only experienced research through their involvement in data collection for medically related studies. With more nurses effectively disseminating the results of studies carried out by other nurses, the value of nursing research will become evident to other members of the profession. The movement away from medically controlled studies has resulted in an empowerment of nurses. Research has therefore enabled nurses to at last feel responsible for the theories that affect the care they give to their patients.

THE NATURE AND STATUS OF NURSING RESEARCH

Research is a satisfying speciality, in that it is not specifically biased towards one sort of nursing discipline. All members of the nursing profession, from general or psychiatric nurses, to district nurses in the community, right through to practice nurses in GPs' surgeries, or even nurse managers or educationalists, can be involved with and benefit from the implementation of research findings.

Research allows nurses to work in a variety of settings. This could be on a clinical trial based on a ward, or as research nurse monitoring physiological assessments for studies planned by public health departments or pharmacological companies. The research may be of an academic nature involved in examining nursing legislation or the effects of policies on nursing as an occupation. Projects can be large or small scale; for example, they could be large surveys or 'snapshots' to monitor the health of the general public, or a small study on a ward assessing a specific treatment for a handful of patients. Research timescales are also not fixed – they can range from a once a week data collection for a small study to a daily collection for a study lasting five years. Research can be undertaken by a nurse either individually or as part of a team, either on a full- or part-time basis. There is also a wide variety of research methodologies: quantitative, qualitative, experimental, historical or even physiological research measuring the effects of certain drugs or treatments on the body's state.

The scope for research within nursing is therefore very wide and is not confined to a particular discipline or type of person or study. All forms will hopefully encourage other members of the profession to evaluate critically their practice and so will help to develop patient care. With so much choice of different forms of studies, experiments or analysis available, the prospect of entering nursing research is a very exciting one.

THE IMPORTANCE OF RESEARCH TO CLINICAL PRACTICE

The most effective form of nursing practice is that which is based on knowledge generated by research. Clinical practice is therefore an important source of potential problems that confront nurses and patients in everyday care. Nurses are in an ideal position to identify problems and can evaluate the effectiveness of nursing practices by, for example, reviewing nursing procedures or by simply observing the patient and the care that they receive.

Research can help to promote knowledge-based practice and so improve patient care. A nurse who is aware or is likely to be interested in what up-to-date research recommends is obviously a nurse who is dedicated to giving her patient the most effective care. Without research, clinical practice would continue to be based on tradition or the hunches of more senior staff. This is ineffective, and at a time where resources are often limited, research can also highlight the cost-effectiveness of a particular procedure.

If you are qualified, then think for a minute of all the procedures that have changed since you began your education. For example, have you found that certain dressing techniques have altered from the time when you were a student nurse? Did these changes come about based on the findings of research? Without research, how would we be able to judge the most efficient way of achieving effective catheter care, or which nursing action is best in improving rehabilitation following a myocardial infarction, or which treatment aids healing in leg ulcers the most effectively?

How can we argue that nursing is a profession if we do not continually assess and update our practices? Research is a means to provide evidence of the weaknesses and strengths in nursing. Without it, objectives for standard settings or quality assurance could not be established.

Research also allows collaboration and increased communication between other health care professionals. As health care provision is no longer isolated but supplied by different practitioners, research can help to facilitate interdisciplinary collaboration within not only nursing, but most health related areas. However, a problem that may arise from this situation is that as research is relatively new to most nurses, there may be difficulties for nurses in separating and identifying nursing problems from medically based problems. Naturally the spheres of different disciplines or professions interact within health care, but only by identifying and recognizing research questions unique to nursing can research within the profession become more valued.

WHAT HAVE NURSING RESEARCHERS DISCOVERED?

Though research is a fairly new subject, an examination of its history would traditionally begin with Florence Nightingale, whose studies influenced health care and, in particular, nursing practice. Her research concentrated on the factors that affected the illness and death rates of soldiers during the Crimean War over 140 years ago. The data that she collected (for example, on hygiene and nutritional status) was advanced for that period and helped to influence the care that the soldiers received from the military. With such knowledge, their level of mortality was eventually reduced from 43 per cent to 2 per cent.[1]

The next major episode within nursing research was not until the 1950s, when research slowly became part of nurse education, especially at graduate level. Interest was also promoted through increased availability of funding for research. It was not until the 1970s, however, that research really took off, when an increasing number of nurses who had the appropriate educational background to carry out research studies appeared and set about enriching and emphasizing the value of research within nursing. It was also at this time that research became part of nursing related policies and documents, and its importance was emphasized by nursing bodies such as the UKCC.[2]

Since then research in nursing has rapidly gained momentum as more and more nurses have become equipped with the necessary skills to become effective researchers. A good deal of earlier nursing practice was based on routine and tradition, and not on the patient-orientated care that is more widespread today. The move away from task allocation towards primary nurse care has initiated more nurses into the practice of critically assessing their work. This shift in attitude within nursing practice resulted in a variety of studies being implemented which have since become regarded as major turning points in the profession. Procedures affecting such elements of care as hand-washing,[3] pre-operative fasting,[4] or even the recording of temperature, pulse and respiration[5] were all scientifically evaluated for the first time.

One researcher who has greatly influenced the practice of nursing, for example, is Doreen Norton and her work on pressure area care. The prevention of pressure sores is an essential nursing activity, but it was not until the mid-1970s that systematic studies into this area were actually carried out. Before this, practice was mainly subjective, with individuals assuming that their own preferred lotion or treatment for pressure sores was the most effective. The lack of any form of scientific basis for this care prompted Norton to undertake three pioneering studies. The first analyzed the relationship between patients' mental and physical state on admission and their risk of acquiring a pressure sore. From her results, Norton was able to devise a scoring system that could identify vulnerable patients who were at risk from such sores.[6] A further study followed this, examining the effects of certain lotions on pressure sores. Treatments at that time were predominantly individually decided, and could range from prescribed ointments to obscure regimens involving egg white, yeast extract or oxygen. Though no particular treatment was recommended by Norton from her analysis, her study did highlight that much of nursing care was based on personal preference rather than on knowledge. Her final study evaluated the effects of regular turning in bed on pressure areas, and the practice of turning patients at regular intervals to help prevent the development of pressure sores still continues today.

THE EXPERIENCE OF NURSING RESEARCH

Perhaps reading this chapter has generated your interest and you may feel that you would like to gain some experience as a nurse researcher. This may be through applying for courses such as the ENB 870, a one-year part-time course offering an introduction to a variety of research approaches, or a masters degree in research, to gain skills in methodology and statistical analysis. However, if you are interested in becoming seriously involved in research, it may be better to gain experience as a research assistant first; many nurses usually become research assistants when first entering the field of nursing research. This is a good place to begin, as it allows the nurse to learn from a practised researcher the processes involved in a research project. Such involvement might also lead to participation in the preparation of papers for the health-related press. It is also good way to learn about data collection and analysis under the guidance and supervision of an experienced researcher. With such a wide range of methodological approaches available, it is beneficial to achieve a good grounding in these methods, which will take time. However this does reduce the risk of a researcher using a particular method because they have had the most experience in it or because it is the simplest rather than the most appropriate.

THE WORK OF RESEARCH ASSISTANTS

Though different projects frequently demand different responsibilities, on the whole a research assistant's role contains seven main attributes:

1. to identify a research question;
2. to assist in the design of a research proposal;
3. to conduct a literature search and review;
4. to design the study appropriate to the research question;
5. to carry out data collection and analysis;
6. to write research reports;
7. to assist in the dissemination of findings.

Proper training in research is essential. As research within nursing becomes more acceptable and more and more nurses become involved in the speciality, there is a risk of projects that are poorly designed, being carried out by unskilled nurses who lack sufficient experience. This can produce a negative effect for both the study environment and potential respondents. Imagine how you would feel if, as a patient, you were asked to be involved in five small studies; each project might be slightly related and therefore it could become very boring to fill in a questionnaire, say, every other day. After a while you might become so disheartened with all this paperwork that you might skip questions or not fill them in as honestly as you may have done previously; this obviously will affect the results. It is therefore much better for the patients and staff if studies are well designed so that there is no danger of 'research overload'. This will also prevent any liaison between a researcher and other health care professionals becoming damaged. If a patient feels unhappy with having to fill in time-consuming questionnaires, then this could affect their relationship, and so will do little to improve attitudes of other professionals towards the importance of research practice.

Some research receives a bad press because of the recent rationalization of health care resources. Managers, for example, may be unsupportive of a project if they believe that it might impinge on financial or nursing resources, or that it might affect patient care, especially if nurses are involved in the data collection. Time is also an important contributing factor in causing some nurses to be apprehensive about the practice of research. Even for those who can identify the benefits of research, inflexible workloads and long shifts often result, understandably, in its being regarded as a low priority.

Attitudes towards nursing research strongly influence its utilization. This may become particularly apparent to new and enthusiastic researchers who may discover that not everyone will feel the same as they do about the importance of research. Recent studies[7,8] have suggested that it may be an overestimation to expect attitudes to alter and research to be implemented unless the environment is open to change. A situation seems to have occurred within nursing, in that it is felt that there are those who do research and there are those who do not.

Reactions to a hospital based trial, for example, may range from enthusiasm and interest to apprehension and a belief that the study is really a furtive way to assess nurses' work. Rettig[9] for example, suggests that one of the most detrimental opinions that exists is that the only 'good' nurse is one that remains at the bedside, and that those who leave this position are abandoning the real world of nursing. This is because there appears to be a divide in attitudes, objectives and values of clinically based nurses and those who are academically based. Such beliefs have created what is known as the 'ivory tower', where clinical nurses feel that those involved in research are out of touch with the real world, and that what they say and what actually happens are two separate things. This may have occurred because of a lack of communication between the two groups: nurse researchers may feel that clinically based nurses are negative and want to remain ignorant about the subject, whilst clinical nurses may feel that academics are not addressing priority nursing problems and therefore they do not maintain an interest in what is currently being researched. They may also feel that the language or layout of research findings alienate clinical nurses from utilizing them, as they feel that they contain jargon or words that are inappropriate, or that they are published in journals that mainly academics would read.

To sum up, research is a systematic method of exploration and investigation, used to solve problems and expand the theoretical base of nursing. It may not be the only way of improving patient care and nursing practice, but it does have a large amount to contribute to clinical practice, nurse autonomy and professional status. The scope for involvement within research is very wide, and with research receiving greater appreciation and value within nursing, it is a very exciting and worthwhile time to enter its practice within the nursing profession.

Notes

1. Palmer, I. S. (1977) 'Florence Nightingale: reformer, reactionary, researcher.' *Nursing Research*. 26(2), 140–2.
2. United Kingdom Central Council for Nursing, Midwifery and Health Visiting (1983) *Nursing Research, The Role of the UKCC*. London: UKCC.
3. Taylor, L. J. (1978) 'An Evaluation of Hand washing Techniques.' *Nursing Times*, 74(2), 54–55; 74(3), 108–10.
4. Hamilton-Smith, S. (1972) *Nil By Mouth?* London: RCN.
5. Nichols, G. A., Ruskin M. M., Glor B. A. K., and Kelly, W. H. (1966) 'Oral, axillary and rectal temperature determinations and relationships.' *Nursing Research* 15(4), 307–10.
6. Norton, D., McLaren, R., and Exton-Smith, A. N. (1975) *An Investigation of Geriatric Nursing Problems in Hospital*. Edinburgh: Churchill Livingstone.
7. Champion, V. L., and Leach, A. (1989) 'Variables related to research utilization in nursing: an empirical investigation.' *Journal of Advanced Nursing 14*, 705–10.
8. Funk, S. G., Torniquist, E. M., and Champagne, M. T. (1989) 'A model for improving the dissemination of nursing research.' *Western Journal of Nursing Research 11(3)*, 361–7.
9. Rettig, F. M. (1980) 'Nurses' attitudes towards research.' *Association of Operating Room Nurses Journal* 31, 1251–5.

SECTION 5
BECOMING A NURSE

You should now be at a point where you are well on the way towards finalizing your decision to become a nurse. You should have weighed many of the arguments for and against nursing, in the light of the information on training and working as a nurse which we have given you in previous chapters. The previous section should have offered an insight into the more long-term goals which nurses set themselves in their career development. If you have completed the exercises which go with the text, these will have offered directions for your thinking in reaching your decision. The final remaining hurdle is applying to the various institutions which offer nurse education and training.

The two types of institution offering courses leading to registration as nurses (the universities and colleges of nursing) come from very different traditions, and their application procedures often reflect these different backgrounds. With a clear understanding of these variations, you will be more able to make the best possible application. Becoming a nurse is now a highly competitive procedure. For example in the universities, nursing as a subject commands some of the highest A-level grade requirements of any subject, and is always oversubscribed. Additionally, many of the universities do not require an interview, so preparation of a strong initial application is of particular importance here. Even where an interview is required, as in some universities and most colleges of health, you have to *get* to that interview, and here again careful attention to application procedure and presentation will increase your chances significantly.

If you do have to be interviewed, a further set of challenges must be faced. Many people find interviews daunting, and it must be said that many interviewers perform the task poorly. Equally, many interviewees come to the interview unprepared. This is a pity, since the interview is a key chance to maximize the likelihood of your being accepted for training. Nursing is about interpersonal relationships, so the candidate who interviews well is giving direct evidence (usually, the only direct evidence available) of her ability to interact with others. As a result, the good interviewee is much more likely to be offered a place. In interviews for university places, a good interview will not only increase the likelihood of an offer being made, but could also affect the level of that offer, with good interviewees being more likely to receive a lower offer.

In this section, the first two authors set out the differing issues surrounding applications to colleges of nursing and universities. It is not possible to cover every practical aspect of application, since these elements vary between institutions but there are a number of general elements which are true for all application procedures. By outlining these, the authors aim to give you a clear idea what to expect when you move through the application process.

An increasing number of people are adopting second careers later in life, and nursing is a popular choice. Although the main route of entry is still as a school-leaver, there are now many mature students both in the colleges of health and universities. If you are a mature entrant, you will find some specific comments about how application procedures differ for you.

Finally, I examine the interview from the interviewee's point of view, so that you will be well prepared, not only to give as good an account of yourself as possible, but also to get what *you* want from the interview, by asking the right questions about how a particular course will fit your needs.

Taken together, these final chapters should put you in the best possible position to become a nurse. As I suggested at the beginning of this book, all of the authors still find nursing a tremendously challenging, exciting and rewarding occupation. We hope that we have helped you discover whether you believe that it will be all these things to you, too. If you have, we wish you well in making your career and choices in nursing.

CHAPTER 13
Practical aspects of applying to Project 2000 courses

Caroline Plews

In this chapter, we look at the practicalities of applying for a place to study nursing in a college of nursing. I discuss the entry regulations and the academic qualifications that will be needed and give an outline of the procedure of getting accepted by a college. I will offer suggestions which will maximize your chances of putting in a strong application which will be most likely to gain such an acceptance. The following is a list of main points to consider at the beginning of your journey through the application process:

- Do I really want to be a nurse?
- Am I too young or too old?
- Do I have the right qualifications?
- Do I know where I want to train?

We will have a look at each issue in turn.

DO I REALLY WANT TO BE A NURSE?

This is a question that underpins the whole of your application process. All educational and training vacancies today are well subscribed and nursing is no exception. As a result of this competition, you need to start with a determined and positive attitude that nursing is for you. If you are strongly motivated this will help you through the entire application process, including any interviews. By this stage, knowing you want to nurse should be something that you can explain to someone; it needs to be more than a strong feeling. Preparation counts for a good deal: find out as much as you can about the area of nursing in which you are interested. Your first stop can be a nursing careers advisory service which will give you some written and verbal information. You could also contact a local college of nursing and arrange to talk to a member of staff.

It must be remembered that some applicants are going to be unsuccessful in their application. If this happens to you, rethink whether you still want to nurse. If the answer is 'Yes', you need to identify what went wrong. Check that you have the relevant qualifications for the colleges you apply for, and have a critical think about the application form: consider how you set about completing it and examine again the suggestions made later in this chapter. Pay particular attention to your personal statement in support of your application: was this as strong as it could have been? It may be a good idea to discuss this with someone who is used to either examining such forms or filling them in themselves. Make sure the person is critical – this is not the time for people to spare your feelings! Check your referees: have you chosen the people who can best support your application? If you did get to interviews, consider your interview technique; it *is* a technique, which most of us have to learn. The more you do it, the more opportunity there is to get it right eventually. You may be able to get feedback on your performance from the college and they may be able to highlight specific areas to improve on. Chapter 15 could then be re-read in the light of this feedback and your own experiences.

AM I TOO YOUNG OR TOO OLD?

There is a lower limit to entry to nurse training, which is $17^{1}/_{2}$ years. However, you can actually put in an application from 16 years. At this end of the age scale particularly, you will need to be able to show that you are ready for responsibility and have a realistic idea of what nursing is about. If you are under the minimum age to start training, you can either continue with education or try to get a job. If you do continue with your education, you may want to consider carefully the course you take. If you know which colleges you are interested in, check to see whether you need any special qualifications, for example a science GCSE. A nursing careers advisory service can advise about relevant courses. Information on how to find the addresses of careers advisory services is given at the end of the chapter.

Alternatively, if you want to find work, then aim for something that ties in with caring for people. For example, this could be work in a nursery, a position as an auxiliary in a hospital, working in a nursing home or a job as a home help. There are also opportunities for voluntary work with a huge variety of organizations and clients.

At the other end of the scale, can you ever be considered too old to start training? Legally, there is no age limit. However, you have to remember that the training is expensive and lasts for three years. The nearer one is to retirement age, the less the health system will be able to benefit from your training; from your 50s onward, this is more likely to be seen as a disadvantage. Nevertheless, I personally knew a student who started her training at the age of 52. Generally speaking, mature applicants, i.e. people over the age of 26, are warmly welcomed by colleges of nursing. There is a recognition that most mature students bring with them an invaluable collection of life experiences, which can be very useful in helping the nurse cope with the complexities of working within the health care system.

DO I HAVE THE RIGHT QUALIFICATIONS?

All applicants have to provide evidence of academic ability. There is a legal minimum requirement, but this can be met in several ways. You will need to meet one of the following criteria:

- 5 subjects passed at GCSE O-level with grades A, B or C.
- 5 subjects passed at CSE with grade 1.
- The equivalent of the above.
- A pass mark of 51 or above in either DC1, DC2, DC3.

The first two criteria are self-explanatory, but I will say a little more about the equivalent qualifications and the DC test.

The equivalence criterion allows candidates to use qualifications that they have which are the educational equivalent of 5 GCSE O-levels or 5 CSE at grade 1. It may be that certificates or diplomas that you have will be accepted as adequate evidence of academic ability. The United Kingdom Central Council (UKCC) is one of the regulatory bodies of nursing. The council has developed a points system for GCSE, CSE, GCE, SCE and Scottish Leaving Certificate. It is possible to have a combination of certificates, and as long as they are in at least three separate subjects and reach the minimum score of 5 points this will satisfy the requirements.

Apart from the points system, there is a comprehensive list of accepted qualifications such as Higher National Certificate awarded by the Business and Technician Education Council (BTEC), Higher National Certificate or some Open University Certificates. Basically, it is well worth checking with the National Board for your part of the United Kingdom, or your local college of nursing, to find out whether your certificates will meet the criteria. An explanation of the points system is also given in the *Applicant Handbook*, which is discussed below.

If you do not have any educational qualifications, this is not necessarily a bar to nurse education: the DC test may provide a way into training for you. This test aims to assess the intellectual ability of candidates in four main areas: verbal reasoning, non-verbal reasoning, arithmetic and comprehension. There are three versions of the test, called DC1, 2 and 3. Many colleges of nursing administer the test to prospective students who lack formal academic qualifications. The test will be conducted formally and will take about one hour. Colleges usually charge a small fee to cover administrative costs, and if you are not successful the first time, you can have two more attempts. Of course, they will be different versions each time! If you are interested in the test you should get in contact with your nearest college of nursing. It is extremely advisable to prepare as much as possible for the paper: the college of nursing will be able to supply you with a guide to candidates which gives you an outline of what to expect. In some areas further education colleges run courses specifically to prepare students for the test. Again, your local college of nursing will have contact names and addresses of organizations that provide these courses.

The above details refer to the minimum requirements, which are set down in law, for people wishing to train as a nurse. Each college can ask for additional educational qualifications. Some may stipulate science subjects or expect A-level passes as well as these minimum qualifications. The acceptable DC pass rate may be set at 55 or higher, according to the preference of the college. You can find details of all the college entrance requirements in the *Applicant Handbook*, available from the Nurses and Midwives Central Clearing House (NMCCH), the address of which is given at the end of the chapter. This book gives details of colleges and which programmes they run, when these start and whether they can offer accommodation. If you are interested in training in Scotland, Wales or Northern Ireland, there are separate bodies that give information for those areas. Again, the addresses are given at the end of the chapter. If you are an overseas applicant you will need to apply to the Board of the area of the United Kingdom in which you wish to train.

WHERE DO I WANT TO TRAIN?

Many applicants will wish to train at the nearest college that runs the course they want to do; personal commitments may make it impossible to consider alternatives. Other applicants may be more flexible, particularly if accommodation is offered. Indeed, training as a nurse can offer an opportunity to move to and live in a completely different part of the country, which is a potentially exciting change to make in one's life.

The *Applicant Handbook* will give you the latest information on college of nursing details. If you are interested in any college, send off for their prospectus and start to get a feel for what they are offering. Students will look for different things in a college. You need to start to work out what are priorities for you, possibly focusing on two main areas of provision: academic and social. For the first, do you want a high-powered institution or a less competitive one? What kind of library facilities, for example, does the institution have, or do they have information technology facilities? How is the course organized? For the social aspects of the course you may want to consider the number of students in the college, or whether there are any sports or recreational facilities. In addition, where do they have their accommodation; are you going to be in the middle of parkland or near a town? It is up to you to decide which elements of the institution are most likely to make you happy.

MAKING AN APPLICATION

Nursing has developed an application system that is similar to that used by the universities. All candidates have to apply through a central clearing house system – the Nurses and Midwives Central Clearing House (NMCCH) – to the college or colleges of their choice. You will be able to select four colleges to apply to. It is important to remember that there is a fixed procedure and time scale for the application process. Applications are processed to cover courses starting in one particular academic year. To be considered for courses starting during this time, you will have to return your application form several months beforehand; the clearing house will give you the deadline date, but if you miss the deadline, your application will not be considered. Your application form will also not be considered unless you meet the statutory requirements already mentioned. It is vital to have all the educational criteria sorted out before you start considering an application. The only exception to this is if you are awaiting the results of exams you have taken. In this case you will have to show evidence in your application that you have taken the exams and then inform NMCCH when you have the results.

At this point your application form will be sent off to the colleges you wish to apply to. Each college will read your form and decide either to interview you or reject you. This is the first potential time for you to be rejected, so it is worth considering how to improve your chances.

THE APPLICATION FORM

Your application form will be read by a member of the college staff who will have shortlisting criteria by which they will select a candidate for shortlisting or rejection. Although these criteria may vary slightly between colleges, some basic principles apply to all shortlisting procedures. First to be considered is general presentation: have you actually filled in the form correctly, neatly and with no spelling mistakes? Most of us are not fortunate enough to be able either to spell perfectly or to write beautifully. I suggest practising clear handwriting and checking for mistakes on several drafts before you actually fill out the form. At this point, be careful not to rush, or to allow your attention to be distracted so that elementary mistakes creep back in. Avoid wasting the earlier practice through inattention at the final stage.

Another crucial area is the space given to you to give supporting information regarding why you want to be a nurse. You need to show that you have a reasonable grasp of what the job is about and link that knowledge to evidence that you are the right person for such a job. Some examples are given below.

Example 1

I am interested in training as a nurse because I enjoy working with people. In addition, I feel that health care is an important and worthwhile job and can give a high level of satisfaction.

At school, I have been a form prefect, and sports captain for one year. Both of these roles have given me some experience of responsibility and organizational skills. I have also worked for several months as a volunteer for Age Concern. In this capacity I helped decorate elderly people's homes and also did gardening. I enjoyed this very much as I found the people I worked with extremely interesting. It was very satisfying to feel I had helped in some way and I gained a lot from talking to the elderly about their lives and experiences.

My personal qualities include a willingness to work hard, patience, and a sense of humour. I do like working with people so the idea of working in a team situation appeals to me a lot.

I have read books on nursing and talked to a nurse teacher and feel sure that this will be an exciting and rewarding career.

Example 2

My previous career was in working as a sales assistant in an electrical shop. The firm went into liquidation and so I was made redundant. Since I have been unemployed, I have given great thought to retraining and have decided that a career as a psychiatric nurse is a tremendous opportunity.

For many reasons it is a logical move. The reason that I went into shop work was to work with people and have some variety. I could never be sure who I would be talking to or what the problem would be. I feel that psychiatric nursing will give the same contact with people but will also provide a tremendous challenge in terms of the variety of people's needs.

I have explored work with clients with mental health problems in the following way. For the last six months I have worked as an auxiliary nurse in a hostel for residents with mental health problems, mainly schizophrenia. I have also done some voluntary work with MIND and been involved in their drop-in centre. I am very excited about the prospect of developing my knowledge and skills in this area.

These examples are just to give you a rough idea. Generally, to sell yourself you need to sound as if you are interested and committed enough to your future job to have found out about what it involves. Being genuinely enthusiastic is a valued attribute. Remember also that the college is likely to be less interested in *what* you have done than in what you have *made* of the experience. The important element in Example 1 is not that the applicant has been a prefect and games captain, but that she is able to explain the relevance of this to her application to do nurse training! Make sure the reader knows that *you* know the relevance of your experience.

The college will write directly to you if you are offered an interview. Advice is given elsewhere in the book (chapter 15) on how to prepare for this hurdle. If you are successful at interview, you will have to decide whether to make a firm acceptance of the place, a provisional acceptance or to reject it. If you make a firm acceptance your application process stops there. If you change your mind, you will have to reapply in the next application period. If you provisionally accept a place this keeps your options open. You may only hold one provisional acceptance at a time, so if an offer comes in from another college you will have to decide whether to keep the provisional acceptance or accept the new offer as a provisional acceptance, or to firmly accept either one of them. Once you have heard from all the colleges, you then have to make a decision within two weeks if you want to accept a place.

At this stage you will have accepted a place, or rejected the places offered, or not received an offer from any of the colleges. This brings us to the final phase of the application process which is known as Clearing. Interviews take place between January and May. The clearing phase goes on from June to September. The NMCCH will compile a list of all the colleges that have places that have not been taken, then send this list to applicants together with a shortened application form. It is then up to you to contact colleges direct, to see whether they will consider your application. If a college is interested, they will ask NMCCH for your full application form. You cannot make a provisional acceptance during this time; you must either firmly accept or reject any offer made.

If you are still unsuccessful, you will be allowed to reapply for the application process at the beginning of the next application period. You will also be given details of your nearest nursing careers adviser, who can help you examine strategy for success next time.

Personal health is an important aspect of your application. You need to be in good emotional and physical health before you start getting involved in working with people in sometimes stressful situations. Nursing can be a tough job, which at times will make heavy demands on you as a person. It is only fair to yourself and to future patients or clients that you have the necessary stamina. If you have had physical or emotional health problems you should check with your doctor or with the college occupational health department that these conditions will not put yourself or others at risk. The application form will ask both you and your referee about sickness and absence rates over the last two years. Having been ill in some capacity does not bar you from nursing, but it must be declared so that a proper decision can be made.

The following addresses will help you in preparation of your application. As mentioned above, England, Wales, Scotland and Northern Ireland each have their own National Boards which oversee the application process for their part of the United Kingdom. They will be able to deal with all enquiries regarding nurse training. They have brochures which will give information about all nursing programmes. If you want to know the nearest Nursing Careers Advisory Service the Boards will be able to tell you. Most importantly they will be able to send you the form to enable you to get your application package which will include the *Applicant Handbook*.

Useful addresses

England: ENB Careers Department, PO Box 2EN, London W1A 2EN (Tel: 0171-391 6200/6205); The Nurses and Midwives Central Clearing House (NMCCH), ENB, PO Box 9017, London W1A OXA (Tel: 0171-6317/6305/6326/6301).
Wales: WNB, Floor 13, Pearl Assurance House, Greyfriars Road, Cardiff CF1 3AG (Tel: 0222 395535).
Scotland: CATCH, PO Box 21, Edinburgh EH2 1NT.
Northern Ireland: Recruitment Officer, National Board for Nursing, Midwifery & Health Visiting for Northern Ireland, RAC House, 79 Chichester Street, Belfast BT1 4JR (Tel: 0232 238152).

CHAPTER 14
Practical aspects of applying for a degree course

Bob Gates

INTRODUCTION

Applying for any new venture in life can be a time of great excite-
ment, but it is also a time that is fraught with a range of practical
issues and problems that need to be resolved. Applying for a degree
course is no exception. This short chapter is intended to give you an
overview of the practical aspects of applying for a degree course, and
also to show you the range of publications and advice booklets that
you may wish to pursue should it be necessary.

THE FIRST STAGES

The very first stage in applying for a degree is being absolutely sure
that you wish to study at undergraduate level. It is important that
you feel fully committed to applying for a degree, and are aware of all
the drawbacks and strengths of higher education; you must therefore
accumulate as much information as possible about degree courses so
that you can make an informed decision as to whether you want to
make such a commitment. Assuming that you have already decided
that you wish to go to an institution of higher education and study
for a degree, some fundamental decisions have to be made: decide
which degree you wish to study for, and decide at which institution
you wish to read for your degree.

The Educational Counselling and Credit Transfer Information

Service (ECCTIS) is a computerized information service that holds a data base of information pertaining to quite literally thousands of courses that may be of interest to you, and may help you to come to a decision. The *UCAS Handbook* (1995) (Universities and Colleges Admissions Service) says that there are approximately 4,000 access points to this service throughout the UK and in British Council offices worldwide. However, should you encounter any difficulty in gaining access to this service, you should speak to your careers adviser, or alternatively seek out a Training Access Point (TAP); these can be found in most large towns and cities. If you are in any doubt seek the advice of your careers adviser as to where these are located. If you are a prospective mature student, the Citizens' Advice Bureau or a further education college or Department of Employment will be useful sources of this information.

Probably the next thing that you should usefully do in the early stages of applying for a degree course is to write to UCAS, requesting their latest handbook. UCAS will provide you with a comprehensive handbook of all institutions in the UCAS scheme and an application form, as well as a range of other current information. On receipt of the UCAS handbook, make sure that you read the sections that deal with: 'Before you apply', 'When to apply' and 'After you have applied'.

If you are a mature student, it is worth noting that UCAS will also send a useful publication entitled *Stepping up: A mature student's guide to higher education.* This short booklet is very informative and I strongly advise you to read it. Although the UCAS handbook is very comprehensive, it is not uncommon for some institutions to forget to update relevant information concerning courses on offer, so always check with an institution that they do, in fact, run the particular course you are interested in applying for. The handbook does not provide you with significant details of the courses that each institution offers, so your next important task is to write to all those institutions offering courses that you are interested in, asking for their prospectus. It is the prospectus that will give you detailed information concerning courses and the institution that run them.

DECIDING WHERE TO GO

Deciding on the particular institution at which you will read for your degree is important, because you will spend between three and four years of your life working and living there. When deciding which institution you wish to attend, you should think over a number of factors that include:

- Does the university offer the degree that you wish to study for, and does it offer the *branch programme* in nursing that you wish to qualify in?
- Do you meet all the entry requirements, or if you have not yet got all your grades do you realistically expect to be able to meet them?
- Where is the university located, what is the accommodation like for students, and how easy would it be for you to get home, for example, if you are homesick?
- Does the type and volume of assessed work compare favourably with other university courses of a similar nature, and do you think you would be able to cope with the demands placed on you?
  It may be helpful to make a list of all the positive and negative aspects related to attending each of the institutions you might be interested in going to. You may wish to consider the following in drawing up your list:
- Do you want a course in one of the new or old universities or a college of higher education?
- What is the host town or city like – does it have theatres, night clubs and good pubs?
- What societies and clubs does the university run; are you able to pursue activities, hobbies and sports that interest you?

EXERCISE

This exercise requires you already to have written to institutions seeking further information about them and their courses. When you have done this, gather together all the prospectuses of institutions that you are interested in going to. Having now thought carefully about which institution you may wish to attend, draw up a list of all the negative and positive factors in attending that course and at that institution. Next identify which eight institutions have the most positive factors. This might well be the list that you should choose as the basis for deciding where to go.

Having undertaken this exercise, it may then well be worth visiting some of the institutions in which you are interested and wish to include in your choices as this will provide you with additional and first-hand information in making a final choice. Lastly, an innovation known as 'Centigrade' is also useful in helping you decide which institution to attend, as well as the course that best suits you. 'Centigrade' is a computer programme that requires you to complete a questionnaire concerning your interests, personal qualities and attributes. The questionnaire is then used to match your attributes to a range of courses and universities offering the relevant courses specified. The cost of this facility in 1994 was £8.50 including VAT and postage. Mature students can take 'Centigrade' at any time in the year from January to November in order to help them make a decision. Students at school will normally take part in 'Centigrade' in year 12 or early in the autumn of year 13. An address is provided at the end of this chapter for anyone interested in accessing this facility.

THE UCAS SYSTEM

The application form

Once you have arrived at a decision concerning the course and the university you wish to attend, next comes the most arduous of all the stages: filling in the UCAS application form. You are strongly advised to read all the instructions that UCAS provide you with before you complete the form. It may be helpful to photocopy the UCAS form and complete this copy in rough, and then, when you are sure that you have all the correct details and supporting information, carefully complete the original application form for submission. Making a rough copy serves two purposes: the first being that any mistakes will only be made on the rough photocopy, and the second that when you send off the original you have a copy of all the details that you have supplied.

You will be required to apply through UCAS almost one year prior to the commencement date of the course that you are interested in, and this should be around October. However, at the present time almost all institutions are semesterizing their academic year and modularizing their courses, which may well affect the commencement dates of courses in future years, and may have implications for the timing of your application. When your application form is returned you will need to submit an application fee.

The application form for UCAS is a four-page document that

seeks a range of personal information about you. The information required includes: your name, address, educational details, special needs, details of employment and a personal statement. The form also requires you to identify up to eight institutions that should be listed in the order in which they appear in the handbook; you should not indicate a preference between them. When pages 1 to 3 have been completed pass the form to your Head or Principal, or in the case of mature students, to your referee. In either case, the person completing the reference should read the instructions for referees. This identifies the sort of information that it might be helpful to include, as well as the protocol for submitting the application form. When they have completed the reference, your referee is responsible for returning the application form, acknowledgement card and fee to UCAS (you should provide them with a postal order to forward). At a later date you will receive the acknowledgement card, to let you know that your application form has arrived.

There may be a considerable delay between submitting your application form and the arrival of the acknowledgement letter, which informs you that all your details have now been passed on to the institutions that you listed as your choices.

Before moving on to discuss offers, it is important to say a few words about the personal statement on page 3 of the application form. It is important to sell yourself on paper. Do not just confine yourself to your academic achievements or aspirations, but tell the admissions tutor about yourself; tell them about your hobbies, interests, voluntary work, church work, favourite authors, travel – in fact anything that makes you sound more interesting than other applicants. It is, of course, best if you can show that these things are relevant to the course for which you are applying! Remember it is a nursing degree that you have applied for, so experience in caring or first aid, and so on, are important to include.

Make sure you get someone to look through your draft personal statement before completing the application form that you will submit to your referee. Remember that there may be hundreds of application forms for the places on offer, and that nearly all of these applicants will have similar qualifications. Make sure your application form stands out from the others. Lastly, the personal statement is very important to you because not all departments within higher education institutions offer interviews and any subsequent offer they make may be entirely dependent upon the application form. When your application form is complete, make one final check for the following:

- Check codes and abbreviations.
- Be consistent.
- Check spelling and grammar.
- Make sure you sign the form.

Conditional and unconditional offers

When your application form is received by the various institutions that you have chosen, they may invite you for an interview to discuss your application. I use the word 'may' quite deliberately, because not all institutions automatically offer interviews, and instead may make their offer on the basis of the application form. The institution will then do one of three things. Firstly, they may reject your application form, in which case they will notify UCAS. Secondly, they may offer you a place on the course that you have applied for, dependent upon your obtaining the results that you have predicted, or that they require (a conditional offer). Lastly, they may make an unconditional offer. This is really for students who already have the qualifications and grades that the institution requires. In the last case the institution will write to you directly. If you are unsuccessful in obtaining an offer, or you do not meet the requirements of the conditional offer, then you will automatically be eligible to go into clearing, and this is outlined in the next section.

Clearing

As outlined earlier, a conditional offer on a degree programme is conditional upon your securing the required grades. If you fail to meet the required grades do not panic. All applicants who miss their grades or did not get a higher education institution offer are automatically sent instructions for clearing and a 'passport' or clearing entry form (CEF) from UCAS. Should you fail to obtain the required grades or passes, you should begin to study the lists of vacancies for courses that you will find listed in quality newspapers on a daily basis throughout September. After carefully reading the lists, you should contact admissions tutors directly, to see if they will accept you with the grades that you have. When an admissions tutor makes a firm commitment to you, then either post or take by hand your CEF to that institution. After considering your CEF, if they make you an offer (and assuming you accept) they will complete part 2 of the CEF and return it to UCAS. Following confirmation from UCAS of a place at that institution, you will no longer be in clearing and cannot change your mind. Clearing may sound like a frightening experience, but be reassured that hundreds of students go through this process every year, and most end up at a higher education institution, albeit not at their chosen place.

I have now explained most of the practical aspects of applying for a degree, the main points of which are reproduced on page 153. The last section of this chapter will explore some aspects of managing your finances whilst studying for a degree. It is extremely important that you think these issues through during the application process, and do not leave it until you are already on your course, hoping that things will sort themselves out.

FINANCE AND FINANCIAL ADVICE

Quite apart from studying for a degree, one of the purposes of going to a higher education institution is to enjoy yourself, and this may be dependent, in part, upon you managing your finances skilfully. A recent study by the Co-operative Bank in Manchester identified that school-leavers underestimate the level of debt that they will have incurred by the time they complete their courses, and this makes it imperative for you to identify a budget that you will work within.

The first stage in identifying a budget is knowing how much you will receive by way of a grant. Your local education authority will expect your parents to contribute to your education, and this contribution will affect the size of the grant your LEA provides. It is worth noting that in 1994 the maximum grant available was £2,560 and the minimum was £1,615 per annum (the grant you receive is arrived at by calculating where you live and what your parents' income is). The whole subject of grants is extremely complex and you will need to get specialist advice from your LEA, as well as seeking support from your parents. Once you know what sort of grant you will receive it is important to make two lists. The first list should be of all your known income and the second all your estimated expenditure. It might look something like this:

Expenditure (£)	*Income (£)*
Rent	Grant
Meals	Sponsorship
Travelling expenses	Parent contribution

APPLICATION PROGRESS

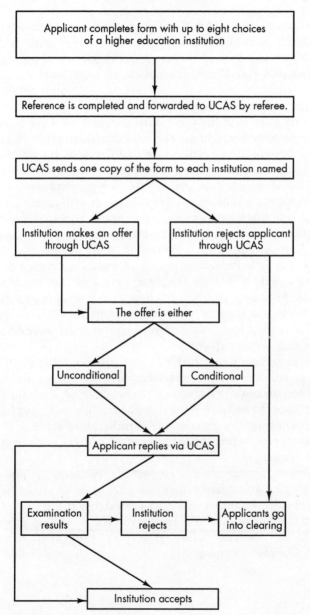

Books   Weekend job
Stationery
Council tax
Insurance

Mature students often find financing higher education even more difficult, because of existing family commitments. Mature students are advised to read section 2 of the *Mature students' guide to higher education* and seek the advice of their local education authority.

When you have made the lists as comprehensive as possible, you should divide your first list (your total income) by 3 (or however many terms or semesters you have on your course) to arrive at a term or semester budget. If you now divide that figure by the number of weeks in the term (usually 10, though semesters are 15) that will give you a weekly allowance that you should aim to work within. You should then total up your second list of all your estimated expenditure, and divide this by the number of terms or semesters and then finally by the number of weeks in each of your terms or semesters; this will provide you with a figure of your weekly outgoings. Needless to say it is important that your weekly outgoings do not exceed your weekly allowance. Once you have undertaken this exercise you will, hopefully, find that you have a surplus amount for each week that is yours to spend as you wish. It might be helpful to look at this as your weekly spending budget and you must endeavour to spend only that amount on yourself.

It is worth remembering that you will still need money during vacations, so part-time or temporary employment may be necessary. You may need to consider taking out a loan whilst on your course. If this is the case, be sure to discuss this carefully with your bank manager or consider the government's student loan scheme. If you are interested in pursuing this possibility an address is given at the end of the chapter.

Finally, this chapter sought to provide you with a practical overview of a range of issues that you should be aware of before applying for a degree course in nursing. As stated at the start of the chapter, the responsibility now rests with you to collect as much information as you can before you make your application to commence a career in nursing.

Further reading

UCAS (1995) *UCAS Handbook* 1995 Entry. Gloucestershire: Linneys ESL Ltd.

Hughes, J. (1990) *School Leavers Handbook*. London: Bloomsbury.

Jones, A. (1989) *The School Leavers Handbook*. 2nd. Edn. London: Kogan Page.

O'Leary, J., and Cannon, T. (Eds) *The Times Good University Guide*. Glasgow: Harper Collins.

UCAS (1994) *Stepping up : A mature student's guide to higher education*. Issue 2. Gloucestershire: UCAS.

Useful addresses

ECCTIS 2000 Ltd & UCAS, Fulton House, Jessop Avenue, Cheltenham, Gloucestershire GL50 3SH; Student Loans Company Ltd, 100 Boothwell Street, Glasgow G2 7JD; 'Centigrade', The Old Rectory, Norwich NR9 5AQ.

CHAPTER 15
Being interviewed

Robert Newell

THE POINT OF THE INTERVIEW

Opinion is divided as to the value of the interview as a method of selecting from prospective students or job applicants. On the one hand, studies from the field of social and occupational psychology suggest that the interview is probably the least useful method of selection, being riddled with personal opinion and prejudice and systematically advantaging certain groups of people (men, attractive people, whites). By contrast, most prospective employers still interview, as do many institutions offering courses (including courses in psychology!). This suggests that there is still considerable belief in the interview as a means of judging who will make a good course member, perhaps as a reflection in our belief in ourselves as judges of character.

Not all courses offer an interview, but many do, and the well-prepared candidate will be able to use the interview to maximize her chances of securing a place. Colleges of nursing and university departments have considerable leeway in the academic qualifications they are allowed to accept from students, and in the offers of a place they can therefore make. They also place varying emphasis on the interview in their selection procedures; some institutions ignore the interview altogether, deciding on place offers solely on the basis of examination and coursework grades or pieces of written work performed for the purpose of selection; other institutions will decide not only on what grades to offer, but also on whether or not to offer a place at all on the basis of interview performance alone. University departments will have 'standard' grade offers, but can depart from these, often dramatically, following a successful interview. In the case of mature students, and people offering unusual academic pathways and qualifications, an interview is almost always required and given the strongest consideration. The task of this chapter, then, is to prepare you as well as possible to take advantage of the opportunity offered by the interview. It is mainly intended for the prospective student on diploma and degree courses, but many of the general points raised are highly applicable during interviews throughout a nurse's career.

Most interviews follow a standard format which involves your being questioned by one or more interviewers, and it is this format we will concentrate on. However, a special section is also included to discuss what I have called the 'experiential interview'. This refers to a series of experiential exercises which selectors use as part (or all) of the process of selecting candidates. The experiential interview will most often include group exercises with other candidates, can be in several parts and can include roleplays and simulations, all of which aim to approximate to what will be required of the student during participation in the actual course of study. These exercises are believed to be more accurate predictors of how candidates will perform on courses, and so be better selection techniques. Since there are so many different possible experiential techniques which might be employed, it is impossible to describe each. However, there are general aspects of presentation during such events which will help the candidate to make the best of them, and these aspects are described.

WHAT INTERVIEWERS WILL EXPECT OF YOU

Broadly speaking, the interview is an opportunity for you to increase the likelihood of your being accepted to undertake a course of education in nursing. As a result, interviewers expect you to come into the interview with clear notions of why you want to do nursing and to be prepared to talk about these notions. In addition, the interviewer will be looking to see if you have the human qualities it takes to undertake nurse education and eventually become a caring professional nurse. As I suggested earlier, it is highly debatable whether an interview is capable of finding out such information; indeed, it is debatable whether such 'qualities' actually exist. Nevertheless interviewers, and indeed the general public, often believe they do, and so it is important for the interviewee to consider how they will respond to this expectation. Interviewers will also try to discover whether you are likely to cope with the academic and personal challenges of undertaking a course at diploma or degree level, often being away from home for the first time.

This is basically what the interview is about, and the interviewer will try and get at this information by asking, more or less directly, about the following:

- previous education and what you have made of it;
- previous non-educational experience (especially important for mature students);
- relevance of these to the course of study to be undertaken;
- why you want to be a nurse;
- what qualities you can offer as a nurse;
- your personal strengths and weaknesses;
- your ideas about the advantages and disadvantages of a job in nursing;
- how you will cope with the emotional and physical stress of nursing;
- how you will cope with the academic work;
- how you will cope with being away from home.

These are general areas of coverage, and may often be asked quite indirectly. As a candidate, it will be useful to you to have thought about these areas and to be able to recognize when they are being asked about.

WHAT YOU CAN EXPECT OF INTERVIEWERS

Fortunately for candidates, the days of the combative, hostile interview are pretty much over. Interviewers are keen to allow you to show the best of yourself; they are not trying to weed out weaknesses in your performance or your academic and personal background. The best interviewers will briefly set you at ease and then explain exactly how the interview will run, including how long it will last and what the structure will be, in terms of who will ask you questions and when *you* will be able to question *them*. Lastly there will usually be some indication of when you will hear the results of the interview and how contact will be made with you. However, not all interviewers are either so structured or so skilled. As a result, some may simply launch into a conversation with you, to which you will be expected to respond. In situations like this, where overt direction is lacking, it is particularly important to bear in mind the interviewer's likely agenda, as suggested above. This will put you in a position of not having to try to fish around in what appears to be an informal conversation in search of the interviewer's intentions. A favourite tactic of the less skilful interviewer, which you would do well to be prepared for, is the attempt to set you at ease by asking some very general question such as: 'Tell me a bit about yourself' or 'Why do you want to do nursing?' Since they are so general, questions of this form often disorientate the interviewee. To combat this piece of interviewer behaviour, have prepared answers ready for questions of this kind, and use them to present yourself in the best light. Although the questions are general, answer them in as specific a way as possible, demonstrating the qualities which you think will make you a good course member and, ultimately, a good nurse.

Many people find this aspect of interviewing difficult, since they are worried about the notion of putting on an act for the interviewer. Rest assured that the interviewer is expecting just this kind of act. Indeed, the skilful interviewer does not place much store by this notion of 'acting', preferring to think of more and less appropriate ways to react in particular settings. Successful interviewees are aware of this need to present different elements of themselves on different occasions, and expect that interviewers will, in turn, respond to appropriate presentation.

BEFORE THE INTERVIEW

A successful interview begins with your preparation. Good preparation not only maximizes the likelihood of your being able to answer questions fully and increases your fluency, but also helps in managing nerves. As a final bonus, good preparation will help you to analyze your performance afterwards and is a source of consolation if you are unsuccessful. Examine the following list closely and use it to guide your preparation for interview, which should begin the day you fill in your application form. Have you:

- memorized what you wrote on your application form?
- a copy of your application for ready to hand?
- memorized/considered the section of this chapter on interviewer

expectations?
• considered the impression you want to create?
• considered/practised some possible set answers to general intro-
  ductory questions?
• considered/practised questions you will ask the interviewer?
• made notes for last-minute practice?
• considered your appearance and decided on your manner of dress?
• decided on your route to the interview?
• allowed adequate time for travelling?

You will notice that this list emphasizes the idea of practice strongly. This should not be taken to mean that you should attempt a perfectly rehearsed set of answers to what you hope the questions at interview will be. A good interview is like a good piece of improvized music. The successful interviewee practises general areas which she expects to occur during the interview, without dwelling on the precise forms of words she will use, just as the improvizing musician practises scales, exercises and musical ideas. The object in both cases is to develop flexibility and facility of thinking and performance.

PRESENTING YOURSELF

The interview is a social event, at which both participants come with expectations based on prior experience. Most selectors, like yourself, regard the interview as an important event, and expect to see some evidence that you share that perception. Therefore consider how you will demonstrate this importance through such things as dress, posture, gesture, social politeness.

Remember that most selectors will be between fifteen and twenty years older than you, if you are a school-leaver. As a result, their interpretation of these conventions may be very different from yours. Seek advice accordingly! You may be concerned that these aspects of social presentation, like the idea of practice, involve presenting a false impression of yourself. This is no more the case than preparing to go out socially. All other things being equal, people who are well presented will inevitably have the advantage over those who are not, whatever the social situation. Interviews are no exception.

CONTROLLING NERVES

Anxiety at interview is, along with anxiety during examinations, one of the two greatest difficulties which students recount. A few students find interview and test anxiety so debilitating that it causes them either to avoid the situations completely or to perform so poorly that their chances of success are greatly reduced. If you are unfortunate enough to be in this position, you need to seek sympathetic expert advice, for which either a careers teacher or a GP may be able to refer you. Reading a self-help book, such as Isaac Marks's *Living with Fear*[1] will also be helpful. Such severe anxiety responds very well to intervention, and fortunately is quite rare when compared with the levels of anxiety which most of us experience at interview. This anxiety can be coped with by the following tactics:

- **P**repare as thoroughly as possible. Good preparation increases confidence.
- **R**ehearse. Repetition of anxiety-provoking material decreases anxiety.
- **A**ttend to your breathing. Fast breathing is a sign of anxiety. Practise slow, gentle breathing.
- **I**nvite feedback on your performance from those you practise with.
- **S**ay coping things to yourself. Remind yourself of difficult situations (including other interviews) you have coped with in the past.
- **E**xchange thoughts which make you nervous for the coping statements you have made up.

This spells out the acronym PRAISE. Remember it as a guide to the steps in coping with interview nerves, and, as a final step, PRAISE yourself for your efforts, both in getting to interview and in coping with the anxiety it will cause.

RESPONDING TO QUESTIONS AND SEEKING CLARIFICATION

During the course of the interview, it is quite likely that at least one question will either catch you unawares or be difficult to understand, either because of anxiety or because the selector has phrased the question poorly. Successful interviewees do not try to answer such questions, since this will lead to vague responses, which are likely to be perceived as lack of competence by selectors. By contrast, skilled interviewees seek clarification by such devices as: 'I'm not sure I quite understand your question'; 'Could you explain a bit more about . . .?'; 'Could you clarify for me . . .?'

Usually this will lead either to clarification of the question or to the interviewer's asking a slightly different question which is less obscure. Bonuses are that it gives you a second chance to hear the question, gives you thinking time, and is perceived as appropriately assertive by many interviewers.

ASKING QUESTIONS, FINDING OUT, AND PRESENTING MORE

Almost every interview will allow you the chance to ask questions of the interviewer; do not waste this opportunity. Many interviewees either do not ask questions at all, or ask bland, factual questions. Consider the questions you ask both as important opportunities to find out more about the course and as ways in which you can show more about yourself to the selectors. It is this second use of your questions which is of key importance in lifting your performance at interview, since, although it appears that you are questioning the interviewer, you are really answering a question which you would have liked the interviewer to ask you, in order to demonstrate some particular strength. You can always find out more about the course at some later stage, but you have only this one chance to impress the selectors. Any question you ask reveals something about yourself, so consider questions carefully in advance and ask the ones which *reveal things you believe improve the impression you will make on the selectors*. Remember also that the way in which you ask questions is important. They represent a final opportunity to make eye contact with the selectors and demonstrate verbal and other communication skills. Be as expansive in your questions as you are in your answers. Practise questions and, whenever possible, avoid referring to notes.

THE EXPERIENTIAL INTERVIEW

At the beginning of this chapter, I noted that there is considerable controversy surrounding the suitability or otherwise of the interview as an occupational selection procedure. As a result of dissatisfaction with the interview, occupational psychologists have recommended the use of selection procedures which attempt to mimic the actual performances to be required of candidates when they eventually begin the course or job. This is similar to the use of auditions for actors or musicians hoping to join a company or band. Unlike the traditional interviewee, the performer is expected actually to demonstrate their skills rather than talk about how well they can act, dance, play the flute, or whatever. So with experiential exercises for candidate selection. Although it is clearly impossible, in selection for pre-registration courses, for candidates to demonstrate that they are skilled nurses (if they were, they wouldn't need to do the courses), they can demonstrate some aptitude for the courses by showing core skills and attributes.

In nursing, these skills and attributes are usually considered to be the ability to communicate, to get along with others and to work with them as part of a team, to examine and find solutions to problems, and to implement these solutions in order to increase client wellbeing. The experiential interview will, therefore, aim to give candidates a chance to show these skills, usually through simulations and group exercises and discussions. These could be anything from discussions of ethical issues related to health care, to practical exercises such as planning care for a patient, acting the part of the cabinet during the Gulf War or planning a group holiday in Devon – anything, in fact, which requires the group to interact and work as a team. Selection exercises can take any time from a couple of hours to an entire day; in consequence the stress placed on candidates is greater than in the traditional interview. The interviewee in the experiential interview is on display for an extended period of time and has to withstand being scrutinized in a variety of situations, usually in the company of others whom she has never met and with whom she is in competition.

I remember vividly the first (and, thankfully, last) experiential interview I attended, the aim of which was to select candidates for a post-registration course in behavioural psychotherapy. The selection took two days and involved the following components:

- a personal interview;
- an intelligence test;
- a group discussion concerning the importance of psychotherapy to nursing;
- several lectures about the course;
- two role-played interviews with clients (performed by candidates on video tape);
- construction of a treatment plan for the client interviewed.

Although the experience was extremely instructive, I remember most the feeling of anxiety which permeated the atmosphere of the two days. Since then, I have used experiential exercises to interview for many courses, and this feeling is always present within the interviewee group. The groups themselves may be hostile or supportive to each other, but the nerves are always raw. Whilst pre-registration interviews are not this intensive, it is as well to be prepared for the atmosphere of tension which will pervade the group on such days.

Apart from awareness of anxiety, how may the candidate prepare herself for such a daunting experience? To begin with, it is worth remembering that, just as in the individual interview, all the candidates are undergoing the same feelings of stress. Second, although you will feel under scrutiny all the time, remember that the observer/interviewers will be looking at the whole group, not just at you. The task of observing group interactions is demanding of attention, and so even the most skilled observers cannot attend to every aspect of every individual's behaviour.

Consider what the observers are likely to be looking for and try to tailor you behaviour *in general terms* to these expectations. This does not mean trying to act out a part for the whole of the selection exercises. If you agree with me that nursing is very much about good communications and working relationships with clients, try and see how these might be revealed by you in each exercise and act accordingly. Not all of us are naturally good communicators, and we may even feel shy in unfamiliar situations like the experiential interview. We can, however, follow the basic rules I suggested for interviewees earlier in this chapter and apply them to the group setting.

Be especially careful to be attentive to others in the group (not just the group leaders/interviewers) and be courteous to other group members. When you want to speak, be clear and do not allow other people to cut you off. Observers will be looking for your ability to assert yourself. Do not be put off if you find yourself hesitating or stammering since this is quite natural in such situations. Remember, it does not matter if you are nervous or shy; what is important is how you cope with this. The interviewer will want some idea that you can cope with anxieties of this kind in the clinical setting for which you will be prepared. By the same token, the interviewer will not expect a virtuoso performance, and knows that some people are more outgoing than others.

By far the most common difficulty in interviews, and in the experiential interview in particular, is in asserting oneself because of anxiety. More rarely, people can have a problem because of being over-assertive. Some individuals are chronically *over-assertive*, riding roughshod over the wishes and rights of others and, as in other professions, there are plenty of such people in nursing. The best of them go on to develop their sensitivity during the course of their lives in nursing and become extremely good nurses, because they are natural leaders. Unfortunately, there are others who are not such a pleasure to work with. At selection, the interview is often trying to sort out people who are over-assertive because of anxiety from those for whom aggressive assertion is a way of life.

As an interviewee, you have two problems here. Firstly, you may yourself be over-assertive owing to anxiety. If so, you are probably aware of this, and it is important to keep a rein on the tendency to seek too quickly, too often and too loudly. In particular, avoid interrupting others and talking 'through' rather than to them. If you find yourself doing these things, an apology will go a long way, not only with the other group members involved, but also with the observing selectors. The second problem is that of being on the receiving end of the over-assertiveness of others. Here I recommend two tactics. First, if interrupted, continue speaking, repeating your point if necessary, and punctuating it with such expressions as: 'As I was saying'. Second, avoid trying to compete in terms of rate, volume and tone of speech. By contrast, when faced with a candidate who adopts a loud, hectoring tone, speak quietly, but confidently and definitely. This will come over as a welcome contrast within the group.

As a general rule, avoid confrontation, however tempting. If carried off effectively, confrontation is an excellent tactic, and will make a good impression, but it requires great control, and is rarely worth the risk in an interview.

The final aspect of the experiential interview is the notion of leadership. Perhaps you believe you have leadership skills. Good indicators are aspects of your earlier life which show these qualities, such as taking leading roles in school and community groups. If you do possess these characteristics, they are important ones to show during the experiential interview, but remember that these exercises are only small snapshots of human behaviour, so it is important that a leader does not create the impression of being overbearing. Good ways to demonstrate leadership at selection include making suggestions, organizing the activities of others through seeking consensus amongst the group, seeking feedback from the group about one's own ideas and the ideas of others, leading discussion without contributing too many of one's own ideas, taking notes, offering positive feedback to others about their suggestions, offering summaries of what has been discussed and decided, seeking contributions from others. These tactics are much less threatening to others than overtly trying to 'organize' the group around its tasks, which can appear domineering.

Behaviour during the experiential exercise

- Remember that you are not under direct scrutiny all the time: the whole group is being observed.
- Consider what observers are likely to expect and act accordingly.
- Be attentive to other group members.
- Do not allow yourself to be cut off.
- Hesitancy is natural and virtuoso performance is not expected.
- Be firm with over-assertive people but avoid confrontation.
- Avoid over-assertiveness owing to anxiety.
- Show leadership skills through:
    seeking consensus;
    seeking feedback;
    leading discussion;
    taking notes;
    offering positive feedback;
    offering summaries;
    seeking contributions.

WHAT IF I AM NOT ACCEPTED?

It may seem strange to end this chapter, and indeed this book, on a slightly negative note, but I want to emphasize that the experience of success is not something which happens to us all the time. The world of nursing is highly competitive and will continue to be so. It is therefore important to go into the initial steps of becoming a nurse with the recognition that at least some of our efforts will not result in acceptance. Since nursing is now so competitive, it is also important to recognize that negative application results are an expression of preference rather than an outright rejection of you as a person.

We all experience let-downs of this kind, often throughout our careers. As an example from my own life, I had had several articles accepted for publication before receiving my first rejection letter. I discussed this with my professor in some dismay, and was surprised that he essentially laughed the matter off. He then gave examples of several of his own articles which had been rejected many times, before eventually being published in highly respectable journals. 'Just keep submitting it' he said; 'eventually, someone will publish it.' And they did!

Of course, the situation of being turned down after an interview is slightly different, but only because we feel, owing to the closer proximity of ourselves to the selectors, that the rejection is rather more personal. Paradoxically, it is this closer proximity which makes interview rejections such a valuable learning tool. All the advantages to be gained from interview rejections can probably be united under the single heading of practice. Let us now examine how practice helps the unsuccessful interviewee gain the most benefit in terms of preparation for the next interview.

First, practice helps control anxiety. You now know exactly how you will react to the stress of interviews, and so are able to pay more attention to anxiety management tactics to help conquer 'nerves'. It may be useful to make a note of exactly what about the interview made you nervous. Second, you know what the interview atmosphere will probably be like, and this familiarity can itself help control anxiety; it also will help in terms of future preparation. You can now consider what kinds of questions you answered more and less well, and take steps to ensure you are better prepared for these kinds of question next time. Use this to target areas to practise if you do 'mock' interviews before your next application.

Similarly, you will have an idea of the actual question areas, and so be able to target these during practice. Of course, it is unlikely that exactly the same questions will crop up at future interviews. The idea is to use questions you have heard at interview as a springboard to help you into the minds of interviewers, in order to consider and rehearse material which you think is likely to be in their minds. Your experience of a real interview can thus be used in conjunction with the suggestions set out at the beginning of this chapter. Finally, once you have had the experience of an unsuccessful interview, the disappointment will never be so great again. Although it is a bad idea to go into interviews expecting to be unsuccessful, the experience of rejection following interview helps to marshal your coping abilities to deal with further difficulties if these occur.

After all this, let me end by noting that the experience of being unsuccessful at interview will surely happen to you at some stage in your career, even if not at an initial interview for a nursing course. However, perseverance is a sure recipe for success, provided we are willing to change our behaviour in response to feedback. Most applicants for nursing courses apply to many different educational institutions, and many end up with a number of possible choices of which course to attend. Provided you are appropriately qualified and experienced to undertake the course for which you have applied, interview preparation and, in particular, learning from difficult or unsuccessful interviews, when applying for nurse education, are principally matters of increasing the number of these potential choices.

EXERCISES

1. Identify friends and family who you think would be good and bad interviewees, and examine what their strengths and weaknesses are.
2. Identify people who will work with you on practice interviews and sign them up to help with your preparation.
3. Work through the PRAISE cycle with regard to any anxieties you have at the moment about being interviewed.

Notes

1. Marks, I. M. (1980) *Living With Fear*. New York: McGraw-Hill.

APPENDIX 1
Glossary of nursing terms used in this book

Associate nurse
An inexperienced qualified nurse, or a student or unqualified nurse, working under the direction of a primary nurse.

Branch programme
The second half of a nurse training programme organized along Project 2000 lines, when the student decides whether to pursue training in adult nursing, mental health nursing, learning disabilities nursing or children's nursing.

College of nursing
An institution offering courses in nursing at diploma level, for which students receive a bursary rather than a higher education grant. Sometimes called colleges of health.

Common foundation programme (CFP)
The initial 18 months of nurse training, during which students experience a wide variety of health-orientated education.

D grade staff nurse
A basic grade qualified nurse, often newly qualified.

E grade staff nurse
A more experienced staff nurse. Often a primary nurse.

English National Board for Nursing, Midwifery and Health Visiting (ENB)
One of the four UK regulatory bodies, which oversees nurse training in England. Similar bodies exist for Wales, Scotland and Northern Ireland.

Health care assistant
A health care worker who assists the nurse. May have only very basic health care skills, or may have undertaken short courses to acquire skills.

Health visitor
A trained nurse, working with families and groups in the community, for the promotion of health and prevention of illness.

National Boards
The four national boards of the UKCC, for England, Wales, Scotland and Northern Ireland.

Primary nurse
A trained nurse with 24-hour accountability for the organisation, co-ordination and evaluation of care for a group of patients in hospital or the community.

Primary nursing
A system of health care which requires that a single nurse be named as accountable for care of a particular patient and, by extension, group of patients.

Project 2000 (P2000)
The system of nurse education introduced into this country a few years ago, through which all nurses are now trained at pre-registration level. This is a health orientated training delivered at least to higher education diploma level and divided into a common foundation programme and four branches.

United Kingdom Central Council for Nursing, Midwifery and Health Visiting (UKCC)
The body responsible for setting the standards for training, professional practice and professional conduct of all nurses. Responsible for all major professional policy-making within nursing.

Ward manager
Roughly the equivalent of the old ward sister/charge nurse. Responsible for management of a ward or other single clinical setting.

APPENDIX 2
Sources of further information

For enquiries about nurse training in Scotland:
CATCH, PO Box 21, Edinburgh EH2 1NT.

For advice about 'Centigrade', a computer matching system for advice about which university course is most likely to suit you:
'Centigrade', The Old Rectory, Norwich NR9 5AQ.

A computerized information service that holds a database of information of courses:
ECCTIS 2000 Ltd, Fulton House, Jessop Avenue, Cheltenham, Gloucester GL50 3SH.

For enquiries about nurse training in England:
ENB Careers Department, PO Box 2EN, London W1A 2EN (Tel: 0171-391 6200/6205).

For enquiries about training and education in management.:
The Institute of Health Service Management, 39 Chalton Street, London NW11 1JD.

For enquiries about nurse training in Northern Ireland:
Recruitment Officer, National Board for Nursing, Midwifery & Health Visiting for Northern Ireland, RAC House, 79 Chichester Street, Belfast BT1 4JR (Tel: 01232 238152).

For enquiries about training and education in the NHS, including training in management:
The National Health Service Training Directorate, St Bartholomews Court, 18 Christmas Street, Bristol, BS1 5BT.

Co-ordinates clearing for college of nursing applicants:
The Nurses and Midwives Central Clearing House (NMCCH), ENB, PO Box 9017, London W1A OXA (Tel: 0171-6317/6305/6326/6301).

For enquiries about training and education in management:
The Open Business School, The Open University, Walton Hall, Milton Keynes MK7 6AA.

For advice about the government's student loan scheme:
Student Loans Company Ltd, 100 Boothwell Street, Glasgow G2 7JD.

For all enquiries related to undergraduate applications to university. Publishes the handbook required when making an application:
UCAS, Fulton House, Jessop Avenue, Cheltenham, Gloucester GL50 3SH.

For enquiries about nurse training in Wales:
WNB, Floor 13, Pearl Assurance House, Greyfriars Road, Cardiff CF1 3AG (Tel: 01222 395535).

INDEX

UNIVERSITY OF WOLVERHAMPTON
LEARNING RESOURCES